RACE YOU
TO THE TOP

THE INCREDIBLE STORY OF TONY CHRISTIANSEN

RACE YOU
TO THE TOP

TONY CHRISTIANSEN with LIZ DOBSON

HarperCollins*Publishers (New Zealand) Limited*

Liz Dobson would like to thank the following people: Tony and Elaine Christiansen and family; Doreen and Bernard Christiansen, Dave Franklin, Phil Hooker, Jim Hainey, Debbie Tawse, Tom Bradley, Janine Ogier, Barbara Dobson, Antony Phillips, Henry and Grace.

First published 2000
Reprinted 2001
HarperCollins*Publishers (New Zealand) Limited*
P.O. Box 1, Auckland

ISBN 1 86950 358 9

Designed and typeset by Chris O'Brien
Printed by Griffin Press, South Australia on 79 gsm Bulky Paperback

CONTENTS

PROLOGUE

AFTERNOON tea is over for the group of financial consultants — it's back to the conference room to listen to another guest speaker during their two-day conference at an up-market New Zealand hotel. The delegates are a mixed bunch — from a scattering of young men and women, to a majority of delegates in their forties and a few cynical-looking men hovering near retirement age.

Some delegates take their seats and open their notepads on the table in front of them, ready for what they expect is another financial whiz touting his company's services. Others mingle around the entrance, still networking; a handful of them study pages of figures left by the conference organiser on a table at the rear of the room. Few notice the changes to the room.

Gone is the large whiteboard on wheels from the front of the room, instead a small aluminium scaffolding set is in its place, spanned by a plank set two metres above the ground. To the right of it a small stage has appeared — the only objects on it are three small blocks of wood stacked on top of two metal stands.

The conference organiser walks to the front of the room and the delegates quieten.

'Our next speaker has a black belt in Tae Kwon Do, is a

qualified lifeguard honoured by the World Surf Lifesaving Federation, is a speedway and race car champion and has a pilot's licence — please welcome Tony Christiansen.'

A door at the back of the room opens and Tony enters. All the delegates turn in their seats as Tony goes past them towards the scaffolding. A couple of middle-aged women nudge each other as he passes. One or two delegates smile as they recognise Tony from his recent appearance on a television current affairs show.

He reaches the scaffolding and climbs up. All eyes are on him now. As he reaches the wooden platform he halts.

'I hope this is Occupational Heath and Safety approved,' he jokes.

A ripple of laughter goes around the room as Tony moves to the middle of the platform.

'Do you know what the first question people ask me is?' Tony says to the delegates. After a few seconds of silence, he answers for them: 'How did you lose your legs?'

CHAPTER ONE

BAREFOOT IN TAURANGA

'As I lay under the train with my legs barely attached I thought, "It's not supposed to be this way, it's not my time."'

I RAN with a big crowd when I was a kid growing up in the then small North Island town of Tauranga in the 1960s. There were ten of us boys that were the same age and lived in a three-street radius — Esk, Harrier and Miranda Streets formed a triangle and this was our domain. And we had everything a boy could ask for in that triangle. We'd ride our bikes and trolleys down the Fraser Street hill, climb trees in the Miranda Street park and run wild in the gully that ran behind Esk Street.

My mates — Paul Hodgson, Wayne and Mark Lloyd, 'Porky' Paul McGill, Gary Winters, Colin 'Snapper' Tapping, Chris Brown, Christopher Smart and Eric State — and I were close and I couldn't have asked for a better group of friends when I was growing up.

We'd known each other since we were little as we'd all gone to the same kindy. Wayne and Mark's mum had turned the basement of their house into a day care centre and the kids in the neighbourhood went there — my mum even worked there as a helper. Then, when we turned five, we boys went to the same school — Merivale Primary — which was within walking distance, so every day my mates and I would walk along

Esk Street, up the Fraser Street hill and then we'd be at school.

I was a typical Kiwi kid — bare feet and shorts at all times, even in winter. I'd play on the jungle gym in the playground and join in soccer games and run around the field with the rest of my mates.

One of the clearest memories I have of primary school is auditioning for the choir. One of my friends decided he wanted to be in the choir because there were some nice girls in the group, so I went along with him. Unfortunately my mate had the singing talent and not me, so the choir teacher, Mrs Dunton, said although I wasn't good enough to sing in the group, I could stand at the back and mouth the words to the songs. I took her up on the offer.

It was my after-school activities that left me with my fondest memories of childhood. The Hodgsons, the Lloyds and the Tappings all had lawns that backed onto the gully, so my mates and I would hang around there a lot.

The Hodgsons' place had a flat back section and a big willow tree that hung over the gully. We boys would climb up that tree and swing over the gully. We'd go down to the creek and try to catch small freshwater herring or little crayfish, but at the end of the creek was every young boy's ultimate attraction — storm water drains that continued for about four streets. The drains were big, but even a boy of nine had to crouch down when running through them or you'd bang your head. Across the start of the drain was a gate with a padlock on it, but that was no deterrent for a kid. We'd regularly smash the lock and run up the drains to the end of them. We were just being typical kids though — the main thing was not getting caught or our mums finding out.

I was always a handful — my mum said that when I was little I would always run away from home. So my parents built a two-metre high fence around the house — but that didn't stop me. I'd squeeze through the hedge and wander away. The elderly neighbours would call out to Mum and tell her I was over at their place. Then a few years later, when Mum and Dad moved to Esk Street and I had lost my legs, the elderly neighbour saw Mum in the street and stopped her.

He said, 'We weren't surprised to hear what happened to Tony.'

Poor Mum, she never stood a chance with me.

Mum, Doreen, emigrated from England after World War II with her parents when she was 18, looking for a better life — not that Mum appreciated being taken away from bustling Harrow to the backwaters of New Zealand, especially as they moved to tiny towns. They eventually settled in the Taranaki town of Okura and it was there that she met Dad, Bernard. He was one of thirteen kids — nine boys and four girls — and Mum and Dad met when the two families got together one evening to play a few hands of cards.

They got married and moved to nearby Stratford where Dad worked as a delivery truck driver. In 1950 my sister Sue was born, and 14 months later my brother Frank. Not long afterwards, they decided to leave Stratford after a horrific crash. Dad was driving with Frank in his little old truck when a car coming in the opposite direction overtook a bus on a bridge and ploughed straight into Dad's truck. The driver of the car died instantly; Dad wasn't hurt, but Frank knocked his head. He wasn't badly injured, but it could have been worse as the car driver was carrying detonators under his front seat. Lucky for Frank and Dad they didn't go off. The accident upset Dad so much that the family moved out of the area to the east coast town of Gisborne, but after a few months they decided to move again as Mum didn't like the town.

Dad had heard about work in the timber industry in the central North Island town of Kawerau, so he and a mate left

Gisborne for a few days to find work there, but they missed the turn-off and ended up in Tauranga. Things turned out well though, within two hours Dad had a job — working for a timber yard — and a house. So he drove back to Gisborne, packed up the family and brought them to the coastal town of Tauranga.

On 23 October 1958 I was born at Tauranga Hospital's maternity annex. A healthy seven-pounder named Anthony Steven Christiansen, or as Mum called me, her little 'afterthought', as Sue was eight and Frank a year younger.

When I was three, Mum and Dad bought the house on Esk Street and by the time I was at school Dad was working as a petrol tanker driver for Shell. Mum left the Lloyds' kindy and got a job as a supervisor at an IHC sheltered workshop at nearby Otumoetai. The aims of the workshop were to enable the intellectually handicapped to earn money by doing menial jobs and to train them to perform tasks. One of their assignments was to cut the points on road markers for the Ministry of Works and then paint a red band around the marker. Mum's job was to help make toys that were sold to shops.

Because of the age difference between us, my siblings and I weren't close. Although they'd tolerate me, I have to say I was a tearaway. I was either at school or at my mates' places and Mum had a terrible job trying to control me. Mum is small, just over four feet, 10 inches, and has a quiet voice, so whenever she yelled out for me I either couldn't hear or (more than likely) didn't want to hear her. So she bought a whistle and she used it when she wanted me to come home. It did the trick though, I could hear that whistle wherever I was in the neighbourhood, and if I didn't come home straight away when she blew it, I'd get a hiding.

One of my closest mates at the time was Gary Winters, who was a year older than me. His dad, Mick, was a member of the local branch of the Lions Club — a non-profit-making group that would fundraise for projects within the community. In the winter of 1967, when I was nearly nine, one of those projects was selling coal. Two wagons of coal had been donated to the Lions and the idea was that over Queen's Birthday weekend we would bag it, put it on the back of a truck and deliver the pre-sold sacks around the area.

Gary and his dad were going to help bag the coal and Gary asked me if I wanted to come. I hadn't done it before, but I pleaded with Mum that Saturday morning to go with him.

The only concern about me going along was that it was taking place at the nearby Te Maunga railway yard, which had the main line going through it and seven separate tracks — a busy place at the best of times. But I was sure I'd be fine, I was going to be with Gary's dad and about twenty other adults. Anyway, it was exciting stuff for a 9-year-old boy.

I remember the reluctance in my mum's voice when she let me go. She was in the kitchen making pizzas and Dad was repairing the fence, trying to thwart our runaway dog.

She yelled out to Dad, 'Tony wants to go with Gary Winters and his dad to the railway lines, what do you think?'

Dad said, 'Yeah he'll be all right. Sue and Frank have been before and there'll be plenty of people to watch him.'

Mum came back to me and said, 'All right, but be careful.'

Later on, Mum said she was grateful she had asked Dad if it was okay that I went as, although she felt guilty enough about my accident, she wasn't burdened with all the guilt of being the only one who gave me permission.

So I took off with Gary and Mick Winters to the yard, but when we got there the parents realised there was a problem. Instead of being on the outer lines, the two coal wagons were sitting on a track in the middle of the yard. That meant extra work manhandling the filled coal bags across the tracks to the truck that was backed up to the outer line. To add to the problem, there was an engine on the second track that was hitched to some wagons and a flat deck with a bulldozer on it. So you either had to walk the long way around in front of the engine to get to the truck that had the empty sacks on it, or you went around the back behind the flat deck.

It was a beautiful sunny morning and we got there pretty early. Gary and I were to get the empty sacks off the truck, take them to the coal wagons, then hold them while the dads shovelled in the coal. The bigger men would carry the filled sacks back to the truck. It was still only about 9 or 10 a.m. and Gary and I went for a bit of a wander — a train yard is an exciting place for two young adventurers. When we came back Gary's dad was very angry with us because we had disappeared in such a dangerous place, so we were told to go and get some more empty sacks. We walked behind the wagons, got some more sacks and then decided to go the short-cut way back, behind the bulldozer-carrying flat deck. We began to cross the track with me closest to the flat deck.

As I went behind it the train shunted — for no apparent reason — with the engine, wagons and flat deck moving back two metres. As the train went back the flat deck hit me on my left shoulder, dragging me under. As I went under I threw my arms out, hitting Gary and knocking him out of the way.

There were dual sets of wheels on the flat deck and they both ran over my legs. I was lying on the track, my legs nearly severed. I would have died within a few minutes after such a horrific accident because of the blood loss, but the wagon's sharp, steel wheels actually crushed the arteries in my legs, cauterising them, so all my blood didn't pump away. But, obviously, there was still a lot of blood lost.

I can remember Gary's dad and another man dragging me out from under the wagon. Of course, I was in tremendous pain, but the shock of it means I mostly remember just being in a hot and cold sweat. As I lay beside the track, I looked up and saw it was a beautiful day and asked for some water.

Gary's dad was leaning over me crying while people were running around screaming. I can remember someone saying, 'The ambulance is on the way' and Gary's dad yelling, 'He'll never make it, he'll never make it.' As I waited for the ambulance, I looked to the side at a nearby house and saw someone running to it. They came back with a jug of warm water and someone dabbed the water onto my lips.

At first I couldn't understand what was wrong and why people were so upset. But I soon realised that something must be seriously wrong and I must be pretty badly hurt. When the ambulance arrived, people were panicking — they were sure I was going to die because my injuries were so severe. It must have been a horrific sight — a young boy, with his legs barely attached and lots of blood everywhere. Their horror must have made me realise how serious my injuries were, even though I couldn't see my lower body. As I lay there I was thinking, 'It's not supposed to be this way, it's not my time.' I knew then, even at such a young age, that I wasn't going to die.

On the short trip to Tauranga Hospital, I fell in and out of consciousness and, according to the nurse in the ambulance, I virtually died two or three times and they brought me back. I can remember her saying to the driver, 'You'd better make it quick.' They had a motorcycle police patrolman escorting the ambulance and I thought that was a pretty funny service to put on for a 9-year-old kid. I still hadn't comprehended the severity of the damage to my legs; all I knew was they felt really funny, all yuck. As we got near the hospital, the cop stopped the traffic at the busy 15th Avenue intersection and I remember looking out the ambulance window and seeing the traffic officer and the cars stopped for me. I thought that was pretty cool.

When we reached the hospital, my parents were waiting for me at the ambulance bay. Someone had rung them up and said, 'Tony's had an accident, he's been run over by a truck, he's all right but you need to go straight up to the hospital.' Mum had just finished a first aid course so she thought about the injuries I could have sustained by being run over by a truck. Imagine what she would have thought if she was told it was really a train! Anyway, as Mum had worked in the hospital as a cleaner, she knew the staff and she and Dad were allowed in the normally out of bounds back bay when I was brought out of the ambulance. I looked up at my mum and said, 'Sorry Mum, but I'll be okay.'

As I was taken into an examination room an elderly charge nurse said to Mum, 'He shouldn't have been in the yard.'

How cruel, as if my mum didn't feel enough guilt as it was.

My parents didn't realise the extent of my injuries and it was only when the well-known and experienced surgeon Dr Paul Mountford arrived at the hospital to examine me that it struck Mum that something could be seriously wrong. She knew it was unusual for Dr Mountford to work during the weekend so she presumed he had to be called in to deal just with me.

It was a chilling thought for Mum.

Dr Mountford came out of the examining room and said to Mum and Dad, 'I'm terribly sorry, but we have to take both his legs off.'

My parents knew the injuries were severe, but not so serious. They couldn't comprehend the situation. Only hours earlier I was running around at home, and now, here I was in hospital with the surgeon telling them he would have to amputate their youngest child's legs.

Mum was shocked at the prospect of the surgery. She told Dr Mountford, 'No, you can't do that!' Dr Mountford said there was nothing else they could do because of the extent of damage caused by the heavy metal train wheels. He told Mum and Dad that he could try to save my right leg, as it wasn't as badly damaged as the other one. But, he warned my parents, the saved leg would cause me ongoing problems and I'd be in constant pain for the rest of my life.

Everything was a blur for me — I remember seeing the lights of the theatre and having this warm feeling all over. Obviously there was a lot of pain, but because of the shock I didn't feel as bad as you'd expect, although I also began to realise that I was badly hurt. Both my legs were run over above the knees but Dr Mountford had to amputate my left leg higher up than my right. The bone in my left thigh had shattered and splintered and was beyond repair. With the technology we have these days, they would have glued the shattered bone in my right leg and put screws in my legs, but thirty years ago, the war mentality lingered — if you had an injury to a limb, cut it off.

The operation took over three hours and apart from dealing with my legs, the doctors were worried about the amount of blood I'd lost. It was a dramatic operation for the Tauranga Hospital staff, as they didn't often deal with such horrific injuries. But I was lucky I had the experienced Dr Mountford. He did the best he could with my damaged limbs, and he did a very good job. I've never had any trouble with either of my stumps; there have been no bone problems, and I haven't needed any skin grafts. After the operation, I think I confounded everyone's expectations by still being alive. There was a possibility I could have died from the shock, from the appalling injuries and from the loss of blood.

My parents went home during the operation and Mum rang the family GP, Dr Fred Martin, who went to the hospital to check on my condition. He rang my parents after the operation to tell them it was over and I had come through it okay.

But he warned my family that I was in the Intensive Care Unit in a medically induced sleep because of my injuries and blood loss. Although it must have been touch and go for a while, Mum and Dad weren't told how serious a condition I was in because in those days they didn't keep the parents as well informed as they do today.

Mum does remember being asked if she wanted my clothes back. Can you imagine it — for a start they were covered in blood and then there was the fact that the shorts were cut. No wonder Mum didn't hesitate in saying no.

My parents, still in terrible shock, came to the unit to visit me the night of the accident, although I was knocked out. My mum vomited when she first saw me — her youngest child with his legs gone. It must have been such a traumatic sight and I know that she still lives with the guilt of my accident.

I remember when I woke up six days after the accident, Mum and Dad were sitting by my bed in the Intensive Care Unit and Mum was still very upset. But as I came to, I felt like I had an itchy foot and went to scratch it. It was then that my mum told me that my legs weren't there any more. They must have been the hardest words she ever had to say. I knew something wasn't going to be right, but having no legs wasn't what I'd expected. My mum then began crying, though Dad remained calm. I was shocked. I kept on thinking, 'This can't be right.'

The next day Dr Mountford came to visit me, and years later he told me he knew I'd be fine because when he came into the unit Mum was lying on my bed cuddling me and crying and I was comforting her saying, 'It's all right, Mum, I'll be okay.'

I spent nearly ten days in the four-bed Intensive Care Unit because of the massive volume of blood I'd lost. I also had problems with my stumps healing. The bandage would stick to the raw skin around the stumps and made a heck of a mess.

So the bandages would have to be changed daily and this was a drama in itself. As the procedure was so painful, I had to be knocked out with general anaesthetic, but I can still remember the pain as they started taking off the bandages. I'd feel really sick as I came around after the anaesthetic and just when I was beginning to feel good again, they'd come and knock me out again! I think I was permanently in a daze during my time in the Intensive Care Unit.

To help my stumps heal I had a bed frame over my legs so the blankets could rest on that, and not my legs. But I was still just a 9-year-old boy in a room with critically ill older people. I would peer over the bed frame and wonder why I was with so many sick old people. I couldn't wait to get out of that frightening place.

The doctors were impressed with my progress — 48 hours after I woke from the medically induced sleep I was sitting up in a wheelchair and when I was moved to the general children's ward I became the quickest kid on wheels. That must have been the start of my racing career.

My parents, friends and family struggled to cope with the tragedy of my accident, and for many days after the operation my mum was in shock. Fortunately her parents, Frank and Winifred, were on hand to offer support. The people of Tauranga also rallied around after they heard of my accident through word of mouth and newspaper articles — the first of hundreds of stories about me. An example of the generosity of the people of Tauranga was when one of my dad's former employers rang up and said if there was anything the family needed, just ask — they'd even pay for me to go to the private Norfolk Hospital.

People's true spirit comes out in times of need.

Although parents weren't allowed to sleep in the unit Mum and Dad's house was only a five-minute drive away so Mum would be by my bedside all the time and Dad would visit every day when he could get time off work.

Life got easier for me when I was moved from Intensive Care to the children's unit. Ward Four had two great nurses — Sister Wesselink and Staff Nurse Howard. They were helpful and kind, and made my long stay at the hospital tolerable.

My family came to see me in the ward and I also had a few famous visitors. Just twelve days after my accident the tall, imposing All Black Colin Meads came into my ward and presented me with a signed rugby ball autographed by all the All Blacks and the Lions team from the 1959 tour. That was a fantastic surprise and a memorable gift that I still have. And word of my accident even reached overseas. Kiwi troops serving in Vietnam sent me a Vietnamese jacket and there was even an article about the troops and a photograph of them in Vietnam packaging up the gift.

Someone loaned me a television — a real novelty in those days — and my parents spent a fortune on the Thunderbird models based on the popular television show. Dad and I would spend hours putting the models together and by the end of my hospital stay I had the whole set of Thunderbird toys. Dad reckons they discharged me because my models were causing too much jealousy among other kids in the ward.

A field officer from the Crippled Children's Society (now CCS) came to see Mum while I was in hospital to see if there was any help or support that Mum needed. The officer knew of a boy with artificial legs in the Tauranga area so she organised for the boy to visit me in hospital. Mum was with me when the boy came in with his artificial legs — wearing shorts! I was so shocked by the sight of these very ugly-looking artificial legs that the boy never came for a visit again.

I made new friends in Ward Four and one stood out, Simon Chase. He was about my age and he had clubfeet. In those days, to fix the condition, they would plaster the feet and make them turn out; and to keep them in place, they would attach a piece of wood to both feet and plaster it too. Simon had to have a wheelchair to get around, so we'd often have races.

One of the worst things about being in hospital — I know it is the same worldwide — is the food. At Tauranga in the 1960s it was horrible — they used to boil the guts out of everything so all the food on your plate was white — white cabbage, white Brussels sprouts, white pork, white potatoes — yuck, I hated it. So one night Simon and I decided we had had enough and would run away — well, in our case, wheel away. Unfortunately, two young boys in wheelchairs were not a common sight, so we only got as far as the local petrol station before an ambulance found us and took us back.

Seven weeks after the accident I was allowed home for weekend visits. Mum and Dad would come and collect me and Dad would pick me up and carry me to the car and plonk me on the back seat. The first weekend visit home was dreadful. Mr Gifford, an elderly chap from Auckland who had heard about my accident through newspaper articles, sent me an old wheelchair to use. The thought was very kind, but unfortunately what he sent was a bathchair-style contraption that really should have been in a museum or an antique shop. These days you'd pay a fortune for one, but in 1967 it was ridiculous. All my mates from the neighbourhood came to see me and there I was in the bathchair with my bandaged little stumps sticking out — I looked dreadful. My mates were dumbfounded and embarrassed and no one would say anything.

The old wheelchair was given the boot after that dreadful episode, but that caused another problem — I couldn't get around inside. Mum or Dad would have to carry me around or otherwise I couldn't move because my arms were too weak to support me and I had lost my body strength from lying about in the hospital. Although she was only tiny Mum usually carried me around on her hip like she did when I was a toddler. Lucky for her I was pretty scrawny then and without my legs I was a lightweight. But Mum wasn't around all the time so I was often left sitting or lying on the floor thinking, 'What do I do now — how do I get around?'

One day in particular stood out for me during my weekend visits. I had been left in the lounge while everyone was outside — Mum and Dad were working in the garden, my brother Frank and sister Sue were out having fun.

I realised I didn't want to be on my own — I wanted to be with everyone else. So I started rolling around the floor and the next thing I was rolling down the hallway. I just rolled over and over on my side to get from place to place. I thought, 'This is pretty cool' — until I hit my head against the wall. There had to be an easier way to get around. So I sat up and started to rock and move forward, but I soon fell down because my arms weren't very strong.

From that day I realised there was a way for me to get about independently. I just needed to work on it and strengthen my arms. So I learnt how to slide around on my bum a little bit and get from one point to another. I soon mastered the technique and got faster and faster and I just moved on my bum all the time — inside and outside. I was so fast that I could move faster than some people could run.

Back at the hospital, my mates would visit me — either being brought in by their parents or coming in with my mum and dad. But Gary Winters didn't visit as often as the rest of my mates. I think that even as a 10-year-old he felt responsible for my accident. I can't remember if Gary's dad, Mick, came to see me. If not, I imagine it would have been because he felt responsible for and guilty about my accident, although Mum and Dad never believed that anyone was to blame.

Unfortunately, nearly two years after my accident, Mr Winters died suddenly from a bad asthma attack. My mum was made to feel guilty about him dying because he always felt bad about the accident. A man even came up to Mum after Mr Winters died and said to her, 'If Tony hadn't had his accident, Mick wouldn't have died.' People can be so unfair.

Although no one was to blame for the accident, years later I did try to find out why the train shunted, as the trains hadn't moved earlier in the morning. I discovered that either there might have been someone up the front playing with the engine, or the airbrakes could have failed. When trains are in a shunting situation, they move back and then they come forward slightly, causing tension between the wagons. So if someone was in the engine or the airbrakes were knocked the train would automatically roll backwards.

Three decades on I can reflect on the accident without feeling too emotional about it, although I do recall the incident as if it were yesterday. In a few seconds my life changed dramatically. The day before the accident I was running around with my mates, playing soccer at school and climbing trees in the afternoon. The next day I was exploring the railway yard, never dreaming that this would be the last time I ever walk on my own legs.

Fate can be so cruel.

Although I can reflect on my accident and my life before it, I definitely have no time for 'what if' or 'why me' thoughts. Sure, my life would have been different if I hadn't have had my accident. Who knows what I could have done if I had legs? But look at what I have achieved without them. I haven't let it stop me getting out there and making the most out of my life.

What the accident did, I felt when I was older, was make me appreciate what I had, not yearn for what I didn't have. But still there were questions. What if Mum and Dad had told me I couldn't go to the railway yard with Gary? What if Gary and I had gone the long way around the trains instead of taking that fateful shortcut? What if it was Gary who was nearest the flat deck and not me? Why did it have to be me?

Life is too short to dwell on those sort of negative thoughts. It happened, and there is nothing I can do about it. I believe we shouldn't use traumas in our lives as an excuse not to achieve our dreams.

CHAPTER TWO
SINK OR SWIM

*'I was the only kid at my school to swim a mile —
and hey, I didn't have any legs!'*

I WAS in and out of hospital for seven months. My life was very disrupted — in Tauranga Hospital, then up to Auckland for tests, then back to Tauranga. And it wasn't just my life that was affected. My mum spent a lot of time with me so Dad, Sue and Frank had to cope in Tauranga without her help.

After my first stint in Tauranga Hospital, I had to be fitted with artificial legs — in those days schools and society weren't prepared for someone in a wheelchair, I had to be like every-one else and walk. So Mum and I went to Auckland to the artificial limb centre to see the specialists and have me assessed and fitted for artificial legs. My stumps were measured for the legs, and then the specialists had to wait for nerve endings and muscles in my legs to adjust to the amputation.

The centre was a pretty daunting place for a young boy — everyone wore white coats and worked in large old rooms. Everything was so alien to me; I missed my friends and family and the carefree life I had in Tauranga. As I was going to be in Auckland for nearly eight weeks, I had to stay at the Wilson Home for Crippled Children. But I didn't like it there as I felt out of place. The home catered for severely disabled children who lived there full time and while I may not have had any legs, mentally I was an active 9-year-old. It wasn't too long before I was getting up to mischief. I made friends with another boy, and we used to sneak out to the local shop in order to avoid the stodgy institutional food served up at the home. We were caught, of course, but you know what they say: have wheels, will travel.

After the assessments I flew home with my mum. As the local newspapers had taken such keen interest in me, a photographer was there to record the event for a story on me. My sister Sue was also at the airport to greet me, so the photographer included her in the photo too. Unfortunately, when the article appeared in the newspaper, the caption to the photo called Sue my brother! She may have been skinny, but calling her my brother did nothing to help sibling relations.

The specialists in Auckland decided my stumps needed time to harden so it wasn't until a year after the accident that I got my first pair of 'rockers'. These were very basic artificial legs made of aluminium and steel and were hand beaten — it took hours and hours for each leg to be made by skilled craftsmen. They were shaped and rolled at the top so they would fit my stumps. The rockers worked just as the name suggested. They were attached to my body around the waist by a metal band with hinges on it. The legs themselves had a rear-facing wooden foot that rocked. To move you lifted your leg and as you put down the wooden part it would rock you forward. Although they were clumsy to start with I soon got the hang of them and could nearly run in those rockers. Of course, the legs were too heavy for me to move by myself so I had crutches, which sometimes hindered my mobility.

It wasn't all plain sailing — or in my case, rocking. Sometimes little kids would sneak up behind me and stand on my rocker sending me tilting backwards and more often than not landing in a heap on the floor. And if the floors were wet I'd slip over as the wooden base of the rockers and slippery surfaces didn't mix.

When I went back to school after the accident I was still in a wheelchair. I was very apprehensive on my first day back. Although my classmates and friends had kept in contact with me while I was in hospital, visiting me and making cards for me, I didn't know how the kids would treat me.

I remember all the kids crowding around me, asking me lots of questions: 'What happened?', 'What was it like having no legs?', 'How was it in hospital?' It was pretty daunting. I just wanted to be treated as I normally was, but I realise now I was a novelty for them and they were just being themselves — curious kids.

Luckily I had a great school principal, Mr Peddigrew, who took a keen interest in me, and a wonderful teacher, Mr Dawson. Although Mr Dawson was a big man, he was very gentle and he made sure that I had a normal class life like any other kid. So in Standard Four I was the bell monitor and that meant spending a lot of time in the library where the bell was. Soon the school kids adjusted to seeing me in a wheelchair and took an interest in me — I didn't have to worry about pushing myself around the school, I had lots of volunteers. This helped me feel part of the school still and meant children interacted with me — I wasn't made to feel special or different. Although I enjoyed school I couldn't wait to get home so I could join my mates and just be one of the boys.

Once I got my artificial legs, my life changed as it was an effort to walk around in them as they were so heavy. At both primary and intermediate school my legs kept breaking down and Mum would have to come and fix them. The metal band was secured around my waist with string tied in a criss-cross pattern. But the string wasn't strong enough and often broke, so I couldn't even stand up with my legs. When nylon cord was invented, Mum began using that, as it was stronger than the string and didn't break as often.

My crutches also used to break down, as they had to support a lot of weight from the steel legs. But the specialists worked out that if they put a stainless steel rod through each crutch it would give it sufficient strength that it wouldn't break. Thanks to me causing so much destruction, that invention was later added to all crutches. Maybe I should make them name the crutches after me.

The first thing I did when I arrived home was take off my legs as they were so uncomfortable to wear all day long. To imagine how I felt, think about what it's like to wear a pair of new shoes that are too tight — they pinch, rub and irritate. Now imagine wearing those new shoes every day for years and the new shoes not wearing with age. On hot days, wearing the legs was even worse — I'd be sweating a lot because I had to wear special woollen socks over my stumps as I couldn't just have the steel rubbing against my skin. But woollen socks and hot, sticky summer days don't mix and the socks would be unbearably hot and absorb a lot of sweat, so I'd have to be careful not to chafe which, unfortunately, I did often. And on top of that the crutches caused chafing under my arms.

Once my legs were off I'd wait for my circulation to come back to normal, then when I finished afternoon tea I'd take off. My mates used to come to my house to collect me or I'd ring them and meet up with them. I'd ditch my legs and instead use my wheelchair or shuffle around on my bum to get about. I could do so much more without my legs on. I could climb trees, and I could even run down the storm water drain faster than my mates as I didn't have to duck.

Like most young boys in the late 1960s I was into trolleys. My dad made me one and I was in it frequently. I also had a simple way of getting around in it — as my mates were dragging their trolleys up the Fraser Street hill, they would tie my trolley behind and drag me up to the top of the hill too. And once you're in the trolley you're all the same — all equal — and I think that was one of the good things about my mates, they didn't treat me differently or let me win because I was 'handicapped'.

Hey, I could even ride a bike. Okay, my mates or my brother Frank would push me up to the top of the Fraser Street hill in my wheelchair and then take me out of the chair, put me on top of one of their push-bikes and then give me a shove. I'd freewheel all the way down the hill because the momentum kept me going. When I began to slow down I'd wobble around, so I'd aim for the gutter then fall onto the grass border. I had a few spills and I can remember many a time when Mum would be standing at the bottom of the hill yelling at me to get off the bike. But I was never going to do that, I just kept on riding.

My sister Sue also let me ride her horse, something that I mastered once I'd learnt how to keep my balance with no legs to support me. But I found anything more than a trot was too much for me to handle — besides, horse riding was too slow for me.

My dad made a shooting gallery downstairs for me in the basement of our house. My mates and I would get slug guns and have shooting competitions.

I did a lot of things the other guys did. It was when they got on their push-bikes and wanted to go off somewhere that I missed out on just being one of the lads. As a 9-year-old it made me feel left out; but my mates were just having a good time, they weren't intentionally abandoning me. While they were off biking, I spent a lot of time at home and I think that's when my artistic abilities were revealed. I'd sit inside and draw on big pads — race cars, dragsters and planes. Those Thunderbird replicas that Dad and I made while I was in hospital started my fascination with models. So Dad and I used to put together planes and boats.

I was determined to do what I used to do before the accident and I was lucky that I had great mates who treated me the same as before and that my parents were determined I'd have a normal life. As they said — I was so outgoing that they couldn't hide me if they wanted to. My parents also instilled in me the fact that I could do anything I wanted to — as long as I got out there and gave it a try.

There is one episode that Mum remembers that proved I wanted to be treated as before. Shortly after I got out of Tauranga Hospital I was playing at a mate's place across the road with the gang when a fight broke out among us on their front lawn. Mum looked out the front window and was horrified to see me in the thick of it. She rushed outside, yanked me out of the ruck and carried me inside our house. Well, I wasn't impressed at all. I sat in the middle of the floor screaming and then yelling at her, 'Don't you ever, ever do that again, I can take care of myself.' I was so embarrassed that she had showed me up in front of my mates, making me seem special when all I wanted to do was be one of the boys. It was Mum's turn to learn a lesson — that I wanted to be independent and not mollycoddled.

At times I was frustrated at not being able to do some of the things that I'd done when I had legs. One day after school Mum called me for dinner but I didn't answer. She blew her whistle, still no reply. Soon the whole family was yelling for me — Mum, Dad, my brother Frank, my sister Sue and her fiancée Doug. But I was nowhere to be found. After a few hours of searching things were getting frantic — I had disappeared. I wasn't with my mates, I wasn't in the house, no one could find me.

Then, out of the blue, I appeared in the house, much to Mum's relief. I was in a tizzy about my predicament so I had climbed up the tree in the back garden and sat there all afternoon. Boy, was everyone angry when they realised I had been looking down at them from my leafy hiding place as they yelled for me and hunted the neighbourhood!

The next day Doug and one of his mates chopped down the tree.

Another problem for Mum was the fact that because I scuffled along on my bum so much I'd wear out my pants all the time. So when the local branch of the Amputees Association visited Mum to see if there was anything they could do to help, she told them about the pants problem. My parents weren't rich people, even when they retired they still had a small mortgage on the house, so they couldn't really afford to replace my pants every few days. As it was, Mum spent most of her free time either making pants for me or repairing them. So the Association came up with the idea of leather pants for me. It sounds all right in theory, but in practice it was a different story. I was the sort of kid to go outside in any weather — rain or shine — and when leather gets wet it becomes smelly, hard and greasy. Very soon the leather shorts were out, but when a local clothing factory started making denim clothes, Mum bought a roll of the fabric and made my pants out of that; and this proved a success.

Despite mastering my artificial legs while being supported by crutches, I was determined to walk on my legs unaided. So I practised and practised. Finally I had my chance to show the specialist at the Otara spinal unit in south Auckland how well I was doing without my crutches. Mum and I turned up for an assessment and Mum told the specialist that I was really trying hard to walk without crutches. The specialist was a bit dubious and he lifted me off the floor, put me on my feet and said, 'Come on, Tony, show me what you can do.'

So, very proud of myself, I took four steps.

The bloke looked at me and said, 'Well, that's not much blimmin' use is it?'

Mum cried all the way home to Tauranga because I'd put so much effort into walking. I wasn't too downhearted about it; besides, I didn't have time to feel sorry for myself — a new challenge entered my life.

When I came out of hospital permanently there was always someone visiting me, usually strangers who had read a newspaper article about me and wanted to help. At first Mum wasn't happy about strangers appearing on her doorstep wanting to help. She even rang our GP, Dr Fred Martin, very upset, and asked him to tell people to stop coming around. He disagreed with her. He explained that as I'd probably live in Tauranga for the rest of my life I'd need these people so Mum should accept the help. Reluctantly she agreed. Dr Martin was right, I have relied on the help of those 'strangers' and friends wanting to assist me. To be honest, I don't know if I would have received all that help if I'd lived in a big city like Auckland or Wellington. I would have received media attention for a while — because of my freak accident and it happening to a child — but I doubt people would have gone out of their way to continue helping me months after my operation. I've always appreciated that about the caring people of Tauranga and when I was older I was determined to give something back.

Two people in particular changed my life and gave a 9-year-old boy focus.

Tauranga swimming coaches and friends of my parents, Dave Franklin and Allan Guthrie, had read in an article that teaching disabled people to swim was a great form of physiotherapy. So around to the house came Dave and Allan with this idea in their heads that physical exercise was something I needed and that swimming would be the perfect answer. The only problem was I hated water, I couldn't swim before the accident and now I didn't have any legs!

It wasn't as if I didn't go near water. My brother and sister would wheel me down to the Tauranga Memorial Swimming Pool that was near our house. They'd be swimming and I'd be sitting on the edge of the pool, flicking the water with my hand, thinking, 'What's the big deal about swimming?' That was as close to the water as I wanted to get, thank you very much.

One beautiful Friday afternoon Mum took me down to the Memorial Pool for the first of my swimming lessons with Dave and Allan. I sat on the edge of the learner pool, which to the average kid was chest deep, but was over my head. I tried every excuse in the book not to go ahead with the lesson, as I hated water. But Dave and Allan were determined to teach me to swim.

My mum was sitting nearby when Dave and Allan grabbed an arm each and threw me into the pool. They didn't ask if I wanted to go in, they just threw me. They decided to use the trusted sink-or-swim method that you use when you want to teach a dog to swim — throw it into the water and it sinks or swims. Well, I sank.

I remember looking up from the bottom of the pool and thinking, 'This isn't good.'

I must have gone under three times before Dave and Allan decided that drowning a boy with no legs wouldn't look good on their résumés, so they grabbed a net used for skimming leaves off the water and just scooped me out. They sat me back on the side of the pool and watched me splutter away.

Mum looked very anxious and Allan and Dave looked at each other and thought, 'That didn't work, what are we going to do now?' My protesting hadn't worked and there was no 'Oh you poor boy, you've lost your legs' — not from Allan and Dave. Instead it was: 'We're teaching you how to swim and here we go.' It was a bit of a character-building exercise for me!

Allan Guthrie was a big man but also a very gentle man — he always gave me the impression of having a gruff exterior, but he was a softie inside. He jumped into the learner pool, with his trousers still on, picked me up from the side of the pool and plonked me back in. My poor mum got another shock — first they tried to drown me and now they were throwing themselves in! But there was method to Allan's madness. He started dragging me around the pool so I could get used to the water and learn to float with his assistance.

From that day I became really passionate about things. Looking back it was a major step, something that changed my life and I have those two men to thank for it. It's so easy to sit there and think 'I can't do that, I'll never do that.' Dave and Allan taught me an important lesson that day about coping with my 'disability' — I had to get out there and just do it.

Allan and Dave knew how to teach people how to swim, but they hadn't taught any disabled person how to swim. So teaching someone without any legs who couldn't even float was going to be a challenge. Starting on that sunny Friday afternoon, I learned how to float, then I started floating around by myself, then I learnt how to swim. Soon one length became two, two became three and Mum and Dave Franklin walked every one of those lengths alongside the pool. Occasionally, when I first learned to swim, I'd start to flag so Dave would have to get the net out just in case I sank again.

I used to get Mum to take me down every day so I could practise and five months after my first lesson — and nearly a year after my accident — I swam a mile, 52 lengths of the pool non-stop. When I swam a mile I was still at primary school and I was the only kid at Merivale Primary School who had ever done it — and hey, I didn't have any legs! For that achievement

Mr Peddigrew awarded me a certificate (which I still have) at my school assembly. It was such a proud moment for me, achieving my first goal and getting recognition for it. Even during that awesome moment I was looking at my fellow pupils and thinking, 'I'm the only kid to swim a mile and I don't have any legs, so what's wrong with these other kids?' Even at that age I was motivated beyond my peers.

And that's why I go through life now thinking: What the heck's wrong? If I can do it, so can you.

When I was 11 I joined the Tauranga swimming club where Allan and Dave were coaches. At the club I competed in races, but I always seemed to be at some disadvantage because I couldn't kick my legs. But I practised — another lesson that's followed me through life and something I still do today. If I'm struggling with something I practise, practise, practise. Soon my arms and shoulders strengthened up and I became a stronger swimmer. My upper-body strength also improved my mobility, helping me walk on the heavy artificial legs with the crutches and also shuffle faster on my bum.

When I got out of hospital, a local solicitor, Ian Morgan, came to my parents and suggested they should make a claim against the railways. They were reluctant at first as suing wasn't in their nature. But Ian convinced them that I'd need some financial support when I was older so he started proceedings. It got drawn out, though, and it took four years until the case reached the doors of the Auckland High Court. I had to be assessed by many specialists to show how 'handicapped' I was. I was examined by doctors, limb specialists and even an eminent psychiatrist to demonstrate the mental scarring from the accident.

I went to Auckland with Mum to visit the psychiatrist and I know he must have been working for my side but the diagnosis wasn't good. He said it was likely I would commit suicide by the time I was 18 because I would be sexually frustrated and I also couldn't keep up with my peers. If that wasn't depressing enough, he also told us that if I didn't commit suicide my disabilities would kill me by the time I was 30. Mum didn't take it very well, to say the least. She had nearly lost me in the train accident and now this important shrink was telling her that I'd either top myself or die because of the injuries.

Her attitude changed, though, when she went to visit my intermediate school teacher. He said to Mum, 'When Tony came back from seeing the psychiatrist, he was roaring his head off, he thought it was funny.'

Mum said, 'What?'

'Yip,' said the teacher, 'he thought this was a huge joke.'

Even at that age I knew that I was going to make something of my life — my injury wasn't a 'disability' or a 'handicap', it was a challenge for me. And so much for psychiatrists' degrees — here I am in my forties, married with three kids.

The Railways decided to settle out of court. I believe they knew that if they lost the publicity wouldn't be good for them so they kept it out of the newspapers.

My case was the last personal grievance claim against a company before the Accident Compensation Corporation system came in, so that meant I wasn't entitled to receive ACC. I also wouldn't be covered — and I'm still not — for wheelchairs, which start at $2,000 and can cost as much as $10,000 for a sports model.

I received about $45,000 from the Railways — that was a lot of money in those days, although, with hindsight, I probably should have gone for more as under the ACC system people were getting $100,000 if they lost their legs. The money was put into a trust and used for schooling and clothing. I couldn't buy clothes off the rack like other kids, instead I had to have tailored pants and jerseys that were reinforced under the arms because of the wear caused by the crutches. Simple things like that.

I had to get a taxi to school every day, which was subsidised by the government. I couldn't catch the school bus because of my crutches and as my dad worked shifts he needed the car. In the end Mum and Dad had to buy a second car, because I had to be taken to the limb centre in Auckland so frequently.

The compensation was also used to build a swimming pool for me. Dad was a do-it-yourselfer and we had a big quarter-acre section so we decided it would be no problem to build it ourselves. Yeah, right. We marked out with pegs where the swimming pool would go and my maternal grandad, Frank, who used to be a bricklayer in England, volunteered to help. My brother Frank and brother-in-law Doug were roped in and even I was out there with a spade.

'If you want a pool, start digging,' my parents told me.

To get a decent-size pool we had to dig eight metres long by three or four metres wide and two metres deep. So we dug, and we dug and by the end of the first day we had dug a square — three metres by half a metre deep. Despite all the sweating and digging it wasn't working. When I pointed this out to Dad, he said, 'Shut up, son, and keep digging!'

But I could see we weren't going to build it by hand. On day two a local drainlayer was called in, along with his digger. With this, a deep enough hole was soon produced, but we still had to dig a soak hole and then lay the concrete. Then Grandad laid the concrete blocks around the side and we painted the walls and put the filter pump in. It was a really exciting family-building exercise.

Once the pool was finished I was in it every day. My uncle owned a dive shop so I got a few tanks and I used to vacuum the bottom of the pool with my tanks on.

I became a very strong swimmer, and I set myself a goal: to compete in the Tauranga mayor's annual sponsored swimming race held by the Lions Club as a fundraising event. I decided to enter the race in 1971 and it was built up in the local papers as *The Boy With No Legs Races The Mayor*. And guess what, on 6 March I beat the mayor, Bob Owens. It was a fantastic feeling and another learning experience for me — set your goals and try your hardest to achieve them.

I also encountered a lot of things I probably wouldn't have if I still had my legs. Mum used to say that nobody would say no to me. I went to Wellington with a friend whose dad worked on the inter-island ferry. I wanted to see how the boat worked, so before I knew it I was on the bridge, sitting in the captain's seat and having my photograph taken for an article.

Another group of people that helped me when I first came out of hospital was the Crippled Children's Society. Even in those days I had a real distaste for the word 'crippled'. The CCS not only offered support for Mum but also showed us that there were organisations around that helped kids with disabilities and that I wasn't the only one challenged in this way. Most of the children involved in the CCS tended to be handicapped through birth defects rather than accidents, so a lot of the kids not only had mobility problems but mental challenges too. That was a bit tough for me when I was younger. I tended to shy away from CCS activities but when I was 14 and 15 I would go to the annual camps held for kids in the small lower-North Island town of Masterton. Those camps were great for me because they helped me integrate with other people with disabilities. These days, I spend all my time with able-bodied people — in my business, my family, with my clients, and now the people who I speak to. But in my teen years it was great to be around people who had the same challenges as me so I could share a lot more things.

At high school my mates were out doing physical education classes and their sports — like rugby and soccer — but I wasn't able to participate in those sorts of things because they were programmes for able-bodied people. When I went away to the CCS camps everything was programmed for people with challenges, and there were people there to help out. Activities were always designed so we could do them — flying fox rides, archery, shooting, kayaking — normal activities that were adapted for us kids with challenges. Those activities were really good for me because they gave me the opportunity to do things that my mates were doing, albeit in different circumstances.

The swimming, coupled with the CCS camps and Mum and Dad getting me out and making me do things, were fundamental aspects in my life. I realised I wasn't the only person with challenges, but also I found that there were people out there who would help — if you asked. That was later reflected in my business — I learned to ask for help. I think a lot of opportunities happened in my life because I asked — flying, surf lifesaving, signwriting. If you don't ask, you never know.

My love for motor racing also started when I first came out of hospital. My dad used to deliver race fuel in his Shell tanker to racing meetings at Tauranga's Baypark racetrack and he'd take me along with him. He used to sit me on top of the cab of the petrol tanker on a little deck chair with an umbrella over me to protect me from the sun. I'd sit up there for the day watching the motor races and I had a better view than anyone else. My dad would be on the ground, pumping petrol and every now and then he'd yell out, 'You all right up there?'

I loved hanging around the track; I'd go around in my old wheelchair and look at all the race cars. I was also spoilt at the track — being allowed to sit in some of the race cars and taken up to the stand to watch the races with the dignitaries. The trips to Baypark also got me interested in racing myself — so I started off with go-karts when I was 12. Some of my mates had them and there was a go-kart track down the road, so I said to Dad, 'We should have a go at this.' Dad made my first go-kart out of angle-iron shelving that was bolted together — the motor was pinched off the lawn mower. When it was finished we decided to race, so down to the track we went with other kids my age and their dads.

When it was my turn to hit the track I sat in the kart and my dad, who isn't a big man, gave it a push to start it. Nothing happened. So he pushed it a bit further around the track. Still nothing. So my dad pushed this go-kart twice around the track and still the engine didn't kick in. We came back to the pit area and Dad was absolutely knackered and was puffing away.

I said, 'Are you all right, Dad?'

And he puffed back, 'The bloody thing won't go.'

So I said, 'Should I turn it on now?'

With that he dropped to the ground, panting, 'You stupid boy.'

Well, that was it. All the parents standing around the pit just cracked up laughing.

Those times were very special for me — I was out doing activities with my dad just like other fathers and sons. I was also very close to my mum, as she spent so much time with me in hospital and then taking me to Auckland for my legs to be fitted. At one stage, just before I started high school, my parents considered moving to Auckland as there were more facilities for me there. They even found a secondary school that would cater for my needs, but I wanted to stay with my friends in Tauranga.

The only down side to the time Mum and Dad spent with me was that, in their teenage years, my brother and sister missed out on a lot of my parents' time and attention that they probably needed as much as I did. They had to care for themselves and although they were old enough to cope, at times they must have missed having Mum around. In later years, my brother Frank moved to Australia and although we don't see each other often, when we do spend time together we are the best of friends. My sister Sue lives near me and we get together when we can.

A member of my family who was an inspiration to me was my grandad Frank. He had a bad stutter and his mates would take the mickey out of his speech impediment, but it didn't worry Grandad. He got on with his life and didn't fret about his challenge. He was my mentor because of the way he coped with his stutter and I was drawn to him. When I was young, I used to do things at a hundred miles an hour. I never stopped to listen to what people were telling me. Grandad made me sit down and listen to what he said instead of running about. We would have discussions and every third or fourth word was a stutter and I wanted to finish the word for him, but he'd get frustrated at me doing that. So I had to learn to be patient — not an easy virtue for me.

I also used to have fun with Grandad. He and Grandma Winifred lived in the small coastal town of Omokoroa, about 20 kilometres out of Tauranga, and I used to stay at their house in the school holidays. The house was originally a bach, but Grandad kept adding more rooms onto it — he was such a jack-of-all-trades. He even built a full-sized billiards table, but then had to build a room around it because he couldn't fit it anywhere else in the house.

Grandad had a boat and we used to go fishing together; these were very special times for me. Every Wednesday he and Grandma would drive into Tauranga in their Hillman Super Minx that they'd owned for years — Grandad eventually wrote it off in a crash. I couldn't wait to come home after school on a Wednesday because I knew Grandad would be there. We'd talk about all sorts of things: we discussed electricity because I was fascinated with it and Grandad explained how it worked; and we chatted about mechanics and cars.

He suffered from Alzheimer's late in life and died in 1997 at the age of 93. It was very sad for me to watch the grandad I knew, who knew everything, turn into this man who was gradually forgetting so much. Once, when Mum and I visited him in the retirement home, he didn't know who she was, but he remembered me. It was a poignant moment, because I felt I made an impression in the life of the man I so admired. But I stopped visiting him a couple of years before he died as he wasn't the grandad I remembered, or wanted to remember. I wanted to remember him as the vibrant man who taught me so much.

American-born **Dave Franklin** *was my Tauranga swimming coach, physical education teacher, and also worked as a guidance and careers counsellor; he was a respected surf lifesaver and won the 1975 surf lifesaving scholarship which entitled him to study surf lifesaving techniques overseas. Now retired, Dave is still involved in the community.*

I remember when Tony's accident happened, as it was headline news and for months afterwards there were items about Tony in the newspaper. At the time I was a swimming coach and a PE teacher at a local primary school, so I decided to get in touch with Tony's family because I thought swimming would be great therapy for him. The only problem was Tony couldn't swim, but the other swimming coach, Allan Guthrie, and I decided it would be a challenge for us to teach him to swim.

Tony was very reluctant to learn; I remember he was sitting on the edge by the deep end — he wouldn't get in, so I pushed him in. That was the start for Tony. He began to make real progress and he joined a class of other kids learning to swim. I remember looking at Tony in the pool — he'd bob his head up out of the water with a big, cheeky smile and water streaming out of his eyes. He was just like any other child learning to swim and it wasn't too long after he started that he swam 52 lengths of the pool. That was a fantastic experience and, I think, a real turning point for Tony. When he was 13 I organised the first Mt Maunganui Harbour swim; this eventually became an annual event. The swim was to raise funds for the Melrose Retirement Village which was being built in Tauranga. Swimmers had to get sponsorship for the race and the largest fundraiser won the Melrose Cup. I suggested to Tony that he enter, but he said he'd only do it if I swam with him. I agreed, so Tony began collecting sponsors. He raised $2,000 and won the Melrose Cup, which he went on to win twice more.

I became involved with Tony again when he started at Tauranga Boys High School, where I was a PE teacher. When the principal discovered I knew Tony, he ensured Tony was always in my PE class, from the third form onwards. I made sure that Tony got involved in sports and organised a special programme for him. I thought Tony would be able to throw a discus or get onto the basketball court in his wheelchair. At the start he'd say it me 'I can't do that' but I'd show him that he could.

About the same time he started high school the local CCS opened a swimming pool at its facility and I organised for Tony to go the opening. Tony got into the pool and showed the children that they could achieve things. It was a moving occasion, especially when Tony took a few of the kids in the pool with him. At high school he had begun to show his talent for art and by the time Tony was ready to leave school I had just finished a guidance counselling course at Waikato University and was back at Tauranga Boys as the guidance and careers counsellor. Tony came to me and said he wanted to be a signwriter, so I approached a couple of local businesses about giving Tony work experience. When I said he was an amputee, they were very reluctant to take him on, but eventually one company did. And to think that he went on to own a signwriting business — it's fantastic.

I also talked Tony into getting involved in surf lifesaving. He was like a fish in the water, no different to anyone else. The only problem I could foresee was getting Tony down to the water, but he either patrolled the water's edge or travelled in the Jeep.

I think Tony achieved so much because of his willingness to give anything a try, the fact that his parents were pretty tough on him, as in they wouldn't let him just sit around, and probably because of people like Allan and I who got involved with him. We got him to understand that he could do something with his life. I'm extremely proud of him and I think he is very inspirational.

Chapter Three
ON THE TEAM

'I had that "no fear" attitude and the blind faith in myself that I could do anything. Ten feet tall and bulletproof.'

IN intermediate and high school I was forced to wear my artificial legs so that I would fit in to what society saw as 'normal', walking on two legs rather than being in a wheelchair. During those school years I was still left behind and excluded, despite the legs. And at times my legs were, and I hate to use the word, a handicap. My mates would be out playing on the field but I couldn't join them. I would have been far better off without the legs, moving about on my bum, but it was more appropriate, the schools decided, for me to wear the artificial limbs. Actually, the schools wouldn't accept me unless I wore the legs and school authorities wanted to send me to Kaka Street school — a facility for people with handicaps.

That school was more for kids with mental handicaps than physical ones, but they said I had to wear my legs or go to Kaka Street. That's what they did in those days — 'Oh, you're not normal so we'll throw you over there, away from society.' Everyone got locked in a stereotype box.

I had to wear my legs right through my schooling. They were cumbersome. They were heavy, they have a big strap around the waist and when wearing them all you could do was stand up and look normal — and what's normal? As soon as I left school, I stopped using my artificial legs altogether.

But the best school plan the authorities came up with for me at the time was to send me to Tauranga Girls College, because it was single-storeyed while the boys' school was on two levels. Unfortunately for me, Tauranga Boys College decided it could accommodate me after all.

Luckily I was with the mates I had had since kindy — my neighbourhood pals — but it was still rough for me at high school. At primary school you stayed in one class with the same teacher and in intermediate the form teacher took you for four or five subjects. But when you go to college you've got a different teacher for every subject. For me that meant going from one end of the school to the other for classes. But the school came up with a plan to keep me mobile. A chair was made for me with handles on either side, so when I was tired other kids could carry me upstairs while I sat in the chair. This was great and the guys didn't mind carrying me either, as the school decided I was allowed ten minutes instead of the usual five to get to each class. So my lifters got out of a little bit of class too. A roster was organised for guys who were interested in carrying me and they also walked around school with me during breaks.

On wet days the artificial legs were terrible — if I slipped over on the wet lino floors one leg would go one way, the other in the opposite direction and I'd land on my bum.

Luckily, I wasn't the only one at the school with artificial legs — one of the rugby coaches had them too.

Keith Empson went through a hay baler when he was young and lost both his legs — one below the knee and one above it — so he used artificial legs. One day he was showing us how to kick the ball between the goal posts but the strap broke on his artificial limb and his leg, instead of the ball, went flying over the post. It was the funniest thing I had ever seen — a leg flying through the air. Funnier still was Keith hopping around the field as he tried to retrieve it. It made me realise that slipping over on wet floors wasn't so bad after all. But I decided a career as an All Black probably wasn't an option.

While the guys were doing physical education class outside I had to do study. I couldn't join them because the school didn't have any facilities or knowledge of how to accommodate me. So I was left to study and draw. This is where I honed my drawing skills and it set me on the path towards becoming a signwriter. But, at the time, I felt left out. During PE my mates would be running around the edge of the playing field doing laps and I would be left sitting in the middle of the field, reading.

Sometimes I think the school unwittingly made me special, made me different. I was often tired at lunchtime because of the effort of walking on the legs. I either spent the break in my classroom drawing or I went to the sickbay and took off my legs so I could rest my stumps. This special treatment was a factor in me doing as many 'normal' activities as I could, to show that I could do things as well as, and sometimes better than, able-bodied people.

At 13, I was strong from swimming and from using my arms to shuffle around on my bum. At school none of the other kids would pick on me because of my size across the chest and in the arms. They certainly never picked on me after I busted my crutch across a kid's head when he teased me! I was certainly no victim and I've always had a 'don't mess me around' attitude. By the fourth form I had a reputation as being a troublemaker. I had a good social time at school but I was never the academic type, possibly because I spent so much time in Auckland having my legs fitted. As I grew, so too did my stumps and I had to be fitted for new artificial legs.

On the first day of school in my fourth-form year my form teacher, Mr Allan Dickson, took me aside. He said, 'Christiansen, a word in your ear. I understand you're a bit of a ringleader at this school so I'm looking for a bit of cooperation here.' He knew that I used to get away with a lot of things because of the 'disability' label.

But, on one teacher, that trick just didn't work.

I was prone to push the boundaries — too far at times — and I found that out in a science class in the fourth form with Mr Andy Campbell.

We were doing an experiment with Bunsen burners. Mr Campbell was at the front of the class, on a raised platform, showing us how to do the experiment. The rest of us were following him with all our burners connected together — Mr Campbell's included. I was a bit bored, so I turned our burner off and blew down it, which made the flames shoot up on the other burners. When the flames shot up on Mr Campbell's burner, they burned the side of his head and his eyebrows. That didn't go down very well.

He yelled out, 'Who did that?'

All the ratbags in my class turned around and pointed at me. No loyalties there!

Boy, was I in trouble. Mr Campbell marched me into the corridor for my first and only caning. And Mr Campbell loved his canes — he had six of them. He had fat ones that didn't hurt but left a big mark, and thin ones that really hurt. He also had different techniques — he'd stick your head under the table and whack you so you'd bang your head as well. Or he'd do cutters — he'd stand on a chair and he'd jump down and whack your bum as he came down. The cane would slice the back end of your bum.

So there I was in the corridor, ready for my caning, and all the toerags in my class were having a laugh and watching from the window in the door. Mr Campbell was going to whack my bum, which meant bending down, but because of my artificial legs, I couldn't bend over very much.

I had to put my hands against the windowsill instead and he gave me a huge whack. Unfortunately for Mr Campbell, he didn't do it properly and the cane hit the steel hinge on the side of my legs. The stick just shattered.

The whole class was in an uproar as his cane split into pieces and I could just about see the tears in Mr Campbell's eyes. So the next minute I found myself in the deputy principal's office looking at a detention because Mr Campbell didn't want to cane me any more.

Another teacher who wasn't impressed with me was my art teacher, Joan Seymour. After examining my work she said to me, 'Christiansen, you're absolutely hopeless, you'll never have anything to do with art in your life.' I wish that I could have employed her when I owned my signwriting business — just so that I could have fired her. Actually, I did have a chance to work with her. When I left school and worked at the Tauranga museum as a signwriter, Joan also got a job there. Talk about karma — her art 'dunce' telling her what to do.

In the fifth form, week-long school camps were held and the options were golf camps, camping and tramping trips, rugby and soccer camps, and photography courses. I was thinking, 'What the hell can I do?' My old swimming coach, Dave Franklin, was a tutor at the college at the time and he suggested I join the surf lifesaving camp he was running at the nearby Omanu surf club. I said, 'Yeah, great. I'd love the opportunity.' The aim of the camp was that by the end of the week you would have earned your surf lifesaving bronze medallion. When you got that you could join a surf club as a qualified surf lifeguard. But to get that medallion you had to learn resuscitation and swim 400 metres in under seven minutes. Piece of cake for me

— I did mine in less than five minutes, two minutes faster than most of the other guys.

We stayed at nearby Mount Maunganui in a motorcamp that had a swimming pool and we used the facilities at the Omanu Pacific Surf Lifesaving club where Dave was a member. He was originally from California, where he was a lifeguard, and he brought those skills to New Zealand.

There were surf skis and surfboards and the other guys on the course helped me get my gear down to the beach. In the water I was as good if not better than a lot of other people because I was stronger. I also had that 'no fear' attitude and the blind faith in myself that I could do anything. Ten feet tall and bulletproof.

At the end of the week I achieved my surf lifesaving bronze medal. So Dave asked me to join the Omanu Pacific Surf Club, which I did, and so began an awesome phase of my life. I stayed with the club until I was 23, when having a young family changed my focus.

But during the days when I worked as a surf lifeguard I had many adventures — one in particular stands out.

One Saturday afternoon my good friend Warren Keenan and I were the two lifeguards on duty in the sunny Bay of Plenty and we were called to a rescue. So I shuffled up to the Jeep, climbed in, and Warren drove us to Papamoa. Three young people were caught in a rip about 200 metres offshore — two boys and a girl of about 17 or 18. Warren swam out to the boys and I went for the girl. She was very upset when I got to her. I calmed her down, reassured her I knew exactly what I was doing and that she was fine. I put the rescue tube around her and we slowly swam back to the beach. She probably had this image of a six foot two, bronzed lifeguard. We got into shore and the water was up to my neck, I had my arm around her and I was dragging her on and we got to the point where she could stand up. And she stood up, and she looked down at me and she looked out at the surf, she looked back down at me — and she fainted.

I gained a reputation of causing more accidents than I saved.

I also attracted attention while surf lifesaving. Many a time on a slow day on the beach during my patrol I'd come out of the water dragging myself along the beach shouting, 'Shark, shark.' That was one way to clear a beach really quickly! Another favourite trick was to sit on the beach and pile sand all around me so it looked like I was buried down to my waist. Then I'd ask some little kid to help dig me out. When they dug down to my waist I'd shuffle to the side and the kid would say, 'Your legs have gone.' So I'd say, 'You'd better start digging.'

When I was patrolling a few people who came along the beach would stare at me, but I didn't care. I was a little bit self-conscious when I started surf lifesaving as this was the first time I publicly showed what I was like without legs. But soon, with the acceptance of my surf lifeguard colleagues, I relaxed and forgot about the stares. In total I saved 33 lives and I received a certificate from the World Surf Lifesaving Federation for my achievement. That recognition was a real honour for me as it proved I was acknowledged for my ability as a lifeguard, regardless of the fact that I didn't have any legs.

I got onto surf club committees and this was a great time in my life as it emphasised that I was accepted by my colleagues. They didn't care about my 'challenges', instead I was acknowledged for my contribution to the sport. Surf lifesaving also gave me fitness and taught me to work as part of a team, especially when I took part in the four-man surf canoe races. I used to do this competitively, which was really great because we used to go away to the carnivals. And more often than not, after a night socialising, I'd be pushed into the motel's swimming pool, wheelchair and all.

I also learned about committing to something and the benefits of training, as well as leadership skills that came in useful later when I owned my own business.

I suppose I was like anyone. If you join a rugby club there is friendship and comradeship, plus the joy of competing. But I don't watch rugby or golf on television — I can't play either of these sports so I'm not interested in them in any form. I do watch motor sport on television, however, because I'm interested in it and it's something I can do well. And competing is something I enjoy, even now. I suppose I am a very competitive person, but my kids think I have to win at any cost. I don't think so. I just like competing and being part of something.

One sport where fair play never came into it was the Tauranga annual emergency services fundraising raft race. Hundreds of rafts of all shapes and sizes would race down the Wairoa River for 6 kilometres.

When I was 17 I entered the race with a group of mates — but we weren't there to win, we were there to cause as much trouble as possible. 'Porky' Paul McGill, Paul Hodgson, Ivan Shannon and I built a raft from drums, lashed together with pieces of four-by-two wood attached with nails and rope. We called it our Portuguese man o' war. We had spikes on the end of our paddles to pop flotation tyres, and knives to cut ropes. When we put the raft in the river we thought we were invincible.

We'd armed ourselves with plenty of ammunition. Porky's dad had a racehorse, so the morning of the raft race we visited the stables and collected fresh manure. It was still warm when we arrived at the river. Ivan had bought a dozen duck eggs four days before the race, buried them in a container in the ground and retrieved them on race day and boy, were they ripe. We added dye bombs to our cache and we were set.

Before the race started we sought out rafts that we'd pick

on — we were ruthless. Local company Profile Engineering had eight to ten guys on a massive raft. If our raft was a Portuguese man o' war, theirs was a destroyer. It had a huge air-powered cannon on the front and they rammed it full of manure, paper, dye bombs and rotten eggs. When they released air into the chamber and fired the gun, it could project the ammo 20 metres or so. It was astonishing. We'd agreed to give a wide berth to this awesome raft but Porky McGill had other plans; he stood on the front of our raft and challenged this destroyer. Bad move. They manoeuvred the destroyer and aimed straight at us.

Porky was standing at the front, with me below him, and he put his paddle up, ready to deflect any missiles. The guys aimed the cannon and fired. The bomb hit him in the stomach and sent him flying off the raft; he landed about 7 metres behind us in the water — covered in cow manure, dye and rotten eggs, and gasping for air. As I was the surf lifeguard it was up to me to rescue him and he was very subdued after that — until we ventured upon the nurses' raft.

There were six women on this and as we paddled past we gave them a hard time and they begged us not to do anything to them. After my many months in hospital, being forced to eat hospital food and suffering the pain of receiving injections, my taste for revenge got the better of me, so we ignored their plaintive cries. We went alongside them, I jumped onto their raft, and pushed each nurse into the water. As a parting shot we cut one of the ropes so a drum floated away.

Our plan of attack on other rafts was to use me as a human cannonball. I weighed 90 kilograms and was very stable as I didn't have to stand up; all I needed to do was jump onto a corner of a raft and I'd flip it over. Of course, my bombing attack didn't work every time, so a few times I was chucked into the water by other rafters. But it was great fun.

About the same time I got into surf lifesaving I also became involved in the disabled sports movement. As a boy I watched the Olympic Games on television and, like many kids, dreamt about one day standing on the dais receiving a medal. I'd think about how wonderful it would be to hear your national anthem being played, with the knowledge that you're the best in the world in your sport. When I was 15, watching the Olympics on television, I decided to set myself a goal of representing New Zealand internationally. Okay, so I wouldn't be a contender for the long jump or high jump, but I soon found out that there were other sports I could compete in. Again, this came about through strangers contacting me and wanting to help me. Once you were over 15 you were no longer under CCS care, so I was looking for something to do because I had a lot of time on my hands. I also knew that there were other people with disabilities who were involved in sports. It was at this time that Peter Pollet and Doug Moore approached my parents about me joining a local group of disabled people who competed in athletics. This came at a great time for me as it gave me a focus, other than just school. I also had the opportunity to learn brand new skills.

Doug was also an inspiration and a mentor to me as he was in a wheelchair — the result of a car crash in the late 1960s — and competed in athletics. He encouraged me and helped to get me to where I was confident enough to compete. Peter Pollet was a hard taskmaster but very enthusiastic that there were young people who wanted to be involved in disabled athletics. He was pushy, but that's what I needed — someone to make me get onto the field and practise after school and in the weekends. Doug and Peter suggested I come and watch an athletics meet that was being held at Links Avenue Primary School, Mt Maunganui — and after seeing other disabled people involved in athletics I decided I'd give it a go.

I started to throw the shotput, discus and javelin, which I'd never done before, and as Doug and Peter knew I was a swimmer I competed in this event too. It was a big commitment, six days a week, three to four hours a day. But I knew that athletics could take me to places that other sports couldn't. I was young, I had an opportunity to see the world, to better myself, and I was also good at it. What enthused me was to the best that I could be.

The disabled movement allowed me to excel in an area of sports that I could compete in. I couldn't play rugby with my mates, I couldn't kick the soccer ball or compete in cycling, but I could throw the discus and javelin, and I could swim very well. This was my chance to do what most teenage guys were doing — competing in sports. Unlike my classmates, though, I was soon representing New Zealand in my chosen sport; however, I always found the lack of recognition for disabled sports difficult to grasp. Here we were wearing the silver fern and representing our country and no one knew it.

I trained for the National Disabled Games in Wellington and competed in wheelchair racing, shotput, discus, javelin and swimming. I excelled in them because I trained very hard and became the best in New Zealand in my grade. In 1972 I was nominated for a New Zealand Herald Junior Sports Award, because of my swimming, but I wasn't a finalist. Instead, I received a letter from the judges — including running legend Murray Halberg and long jump champion Yvette Corlett — saying they were impressed with my 'courage and determination'.

'We feel sure that no matter how big the task, you will do well. Such courage as you have shown must surely meet its due reward,' the judges' letter said.

That was a real honour for me.

So while my mates were out doing rugby training I was

out doing my training and I became very sports-oriented. After the 1975 nationals we waited four weeks before they announced the team for the Far Eastern and South Pacific Games for the Handicapped (FESPIC) in Oita, Japan, and it was an anxious time for me. I was in the basement of our house when the telephone call came through from the selectors. I can remember coming up the spiral staircase that led from our basement, and Mum met me at the top and told me that I was in the team. That was a very special moment for me, because I was only 16. We left for Japan a month after the team was announced, but before then I had to get all my injections and organise all the things that were needed for the trip — like my passport and clothing. I remember meeting the team in Auckland before we flew out. I was very excited because it was my first time representing New Zealand and I was the youngest team member. Several of the older, experienced guys in the team befriended me and even gave me a nickname — Flipper. I earned this because I was good swimmer and always in the pool, and also when I ran around the pool in my wet swimming trunks they would flip-flop on the ground.

I remember the excitement of being on the plane with the team — it was the first time I'd been overseas and my first time on such a large aircraft. We were seated at the back of the plane because that was where they loaded all the wheelchairs on. The team sat together and we were having a great time. The older members of the team were drinking alcohol; I was too young to, but I was climbing on the back of seats and 'yahooing', making a nuisance of myself. My team mates egged me on, but unfortunately the cabin crew were less impressed with my behaviour and one of the flight attendants said to me, 'Why don't you go outside and play?'

That joke stuck with me and the people in the team for many years.

We stopped in Hong Kong overnight and that was a massive eye-opener for me — I certainly wasn't in Tauranga any more! I was pretty blown away by the hustle and bustle of the place, the fast pace of the people and the neverending traffic. A group of us in wheelchairs decided to go for a quick sightsee and that was another remarkable adventure for me. For a start it was hard to get around — the footpaths were being dug up around shop fronts and we had to contend with the constant flow of people who had no regard for a group of Kiwis in wheelchairs. I'm sure we got our fair share of stares from the locals.

I couldn't get over the humidity of Hong Kong and the totally different lifestyle compared to my existence in Tauranga. No houses on quarter-acre sections — instead there were highrise apartments and shanty blocks. The traffic also blew me away — in Tauranga we still didn't have any traffic lights and there was one main street, Cameron Road. In Hong Kong, there was every imaginable mode of transport.

I had decided to buy a watch and a car stereo for my new car while I was in Hong Kong, as they were cheaper there than in New Zealand and at the time there wasn't a wide range of stereos available at home. Friends at home had told me which brand of stereo to look out for, so while I was sightseeing we checked out duty free shops and I planned to buy my goods during our three-day stopover on the way home from the Games.

The flight to Japan was uneventful — I had learnt my lesson on the way to Hong Kong and decided to behave — no in-flight entertainment from Tony Christiansen, thank you very much. When we landed at Oita, the venue for the Games, I was blown away by the reception. There were school children waiting to greet us, bands playing and an official welcoming party.

That was my first realisation that I had achieved my dream

— there I was, representing my country overseas.

They took us by bus to the Games village — a massive apartment block — across the road from the stadium. In the next few days we trained and acclimatised. It felt fantastic to be involved in the team and at times I couldn't believe my good fortune.

The FESPIC Games were from 1–3 June and the opening ceremony was incredible. There were 40,000 people in the stadium watching the event and as I wheeled around the stadium I was awestruck by the surroundings. Here I was, Tony Christiansen from Tauranga, in front of a huge crowd in Oita, Japan. I felt very proud in my team uniform with the silver fern on it. I'm sure all sportspeople must feel this way when they make it to an international event.

Unlike the able-bodied Olympic competitors, we competed in many events. I represented New Zealand in the shotput, discus, javelin, wheelchair racing in the 100 and 400 metres, pentathlon and the swimming events. That also meant you tended to compete against the same guys in every event. Those fellow competitors gave me the nickname Kiwi and they were a supportive bunch. As I was competing in the 100 metre sprint I was running third when I heard the guys in the next heat yelling out, 'Go, Kiwi!' That spurred me on; I won my heat, and then went on to come second in the final. When I won the silver medal the officials called me up and I sat in my wheelchair in front of the dais. I felt deeply honoured when the official slipped the medal over my neck and shook my hand. When they played the New Zealand anthem, I had a tear in my eye. It was a moving experience that will always live with me. Life doesn't get much better than this. I had set a goal to represent New Zealand, trained hard and finally won a medal. Awesome. After dreaming about winning a medal when I was a young boy, the real experience was better than I ever imagined.

I went on to win gold in the swimming and javelin.

During the Games each competitor was assigned an interpreter, usually a student learning English at the local college. They stayed with us during the day and worked as a helper. Part of our job in return was to teach them better English. My interpreter was an attractive young woman called Yumiko and I got on very well with her. She showed me the sights of Oita and I socialised with her, too, at the many evening functions held during the Games.

The event wasn't just about competing, it was about friendships and bonding with other people around the world with challenges who were also striving to be the best in their sport.

One of the funniest incidents I can remember about the Games, away from the events, happened at the village. I was going back to my room in the apartment block with my team mate and friend Paul Curry, who shared the room with me. We got into the lift and told the lift operator which floor we wanted and as the doors were about to close the captain of the Australian team, an able-bodied guy, got into the lift with us. He made it very obvious he was in a hurry when he told the operator which floor he needed. So you can imagine his reaction when the lift missed his destination. He wasn't impressed, and he let fly with a stream of abuse at the young female lift operator. He had a thick Aussie accent and he swore at her for getting the floors wrong. The lift operator just looked at him and smiled and didn't say a word. Eventually the lift arrived at his floor and the unpleasant gentleman got out. As the doors to the lift shut, the operator turned to us and said in perfect English, 'Not a very pleasant person, was he?' Paul and I laughed. There we were thinking that she didn't understand a word of the abuse hurled at her, when in reality she did, but just ignored the pompous man. I'll never forget that incident. Lift Operator 1, Australia 0.

On the way home we stopped in Hong Kong for three days and stayed at the YMCA. I had a room on the fourteenth floor that had a great view of the city. You looked out over the top of surrounding buildings that were nothing more than slum blocks. From the front they looked fine, but when you looked at the back you saw how run down they were, with leaking air conditioning units on the side of the apartment buildings. I could see people living on roofs and under canopies, and it was an eye-opener for me.

After some retail therapy and souvenir hunting, and purchasing my watch and car stereo, we did some more sightseeing. We went for a tour to the Chinese border and looked out from a plateau across to China. Although the sight was magnificent, it was also a sobering experience as the guide explained to us about people trying to escape from China into Hong Kong. Ten thousand people a year tried to get across the border and only two usually made it. What happened to the unsuccessful ones, the guide said, wasn't known. We tried to spot the border guards but we couldn't see a single soul; then the guide told us that the soldiers were hidden in tunnels.

It was a solemn encounter with another way of life, especially for me as I was younger than the rest of the team and never really imagined anything like that happened in the world. It certainly made me appreciate my life in Tauranga and in some way made me determined to make the most of my circumstances, no matter what.

Representing New Zealand that first time was a phenomenal achievement for me. It showed me what motivation could do. It also proved that you should dream; and, if you tried hard enough, you could achieve that dream.

In 1976 I was a finalist in the Herald's Sports Awards because of my achievement at FESPIC; I felt I had received recognition for my hours of training that led me to be the best in the world in my field. I went on to represent New Zealand five times at the World, FESPIC and Paralympics Games, winning thirty-five medals — twelve gold, seventeen silver and six bronze — during my athletics career.

My sports took me around the world — to Japan, Canada, Hong Kong, and twice to Australia. Every time I represented New Zealand was a special occasion, and every time I won a medal I celebrated because I had striven to be the best — and succeeded.

In 1977 I competed in the FESPIC Games in Sydney and won gold in the shotput, discus, javelin, pentathlon, and 100 metre swim; silver in the 50 metre freestyle and bronze in snooker. Based on my results I was voted best amputee competitor of the Games by the organisers. Unfortunately, I wasn't able to accept the award myself as I was still competing in the pentathlon and was in-between venues. But the manager of the New Zealand team accepted it for me and presented it to me that night. It was a real honour for me to be nominated for the award as there were so many other talented athletes.

I was especially pleased with my results as, because of a rule change, this was the first FESPIC Games in which I competed against a person with one leg. I was graded B2, an amputee grade, but the one-legged competitor was in the same grade as me because the rules didn't differentiate between standing or sitting. This meant he was at an advantage when competing and this stood out in the javelin as he was able to hop in his circle — the standard two-metre diameter circle — while I was seated in the chair circle. The chair that you throw from is strapped down to the ground so the throwing position is always sitting. It was easy to see the advantage he had from having the extra height and being able to move in his circle. He could get some momentum and his best flights were better than mine, but as he wasn't able to use his artificial leg, he had problems with his balance. One of his better throws beat mine, but he fell over outside the circle and the throw was disqualified.

After the 1977 FESPIC Games the grading was changed so a double amputee didn't have to compete against a single amputee.

Aside from competing, one of the important things I remember about the 1977 Games was my friendship with another New Zealand team member, Brian Portland. Brian and I were very similar, in many ways. He lost both his legs in a shunting accident when he was working at a railway yard, after he was caught between two carriages. Our amputations were basically the same, although our long stumps were on opposite sides. Brian was about ten years older than me and for some reason people thought we were brothers or twins because we were both in wheelchairs, both had legs amputated and we hung around together. At the Games we bunked together and there was a rivalry between us. I later found out that at one of my events Brian had a side bet with someone and he bet against me — but I won. All those things were taken in good fun.

World competition is real competition. It doesn't matter where you are competing, each person is your rival, they are out to best you, whatever you've done. You wouldn't be there if you hadn't reached a qualifying standard. So everyone who I competed against was of the same quality and same standard as I was. There was intensity in the finals because this was the culmination of months of training.

Even though the 'disabled' competitions were notable for the comradeship and friendships that formed, once you were on the field, it didn't matter who you were or what you were, or what you'd had cut off — you were just another rival.

The achievements of other competitors were an eye-opener for me. I knew the background of the other New Zealand competitors and what they were doing, but when I was competing overseas I was introduced to an amazing group of athletes. For instance, the Olympic high jumpers with one leg were jumping just centimetres below able-bodied record holders. And to see Olympic blind runners competing in the 100 metre sprint was amazing. They would sprint by themselves with just a helper at the end of the track yelling directions to them like 'straight ahead', 'left', 'right', or ringing a bell. It was inspiring for me — the faith that the blind runners had in the person at the other end of the track was tremendous. People call what I have achieved amazing, but when I saw other competitors it was I who was amazed by what people have done.

Although all the international events were extraordinary, there was one that stood out the most for me — the 1980 Paralympics in Holland.

It was the final of the 100 metre backstroke. When I was getting into the pool with the other competitors, I looked across to the side as they lifted a young man from Israel out of his wheelchair and into the pool. He had spina bifida and had short, twisted arms, a very short body and little legs. But that didn't stop him trying and when the race started he began floating on his back. I finished second in a time of just under 70 seconds. We got out of the pool, dried ourselves and then we looked back into the pool — the little man was still going. His arms were flipping away and now and then he'd sink under the water and come back up and spit the water out.

It took him nine minutes to finish the event.

We were up on the podium, receiving our medals and hearing our national anthems being played. It was a very proud moment for me and as moving as I'd always imagined it would be. But it was a prouder moment when we three finalists took off our medals and offered them to the young Israeli man. We felt his achievement was greater than ours — we'd won the race, and that's what we'd trained for, but he finished.

In 1980 I was selected to represent New Zealand at the Canadian amputee national championships in Vancouver. The newly established New Zealand Amputee Sports Association had been invited to send a team to attend the championships. The association had been created as many amputees hadn't been selected for the next Paralympics. It was felt the national paraplegic sports body wasn't catering for the promotion of amputees, and was selecting other disabled people ahead of them.

A team of five, plus a manager, attended the Canadian championships and I competed in the shotput, discus and javelin, plus swimming and a few wheelchair races. I also competed in pentathlon — shotput, javelin, swimming, wheelchair racing and rifle shooting. I hadn't quite mastered shooting, so it was great when I won the silver medal.

It was a great group of guys I went to Canada with — there were two of us in wheelchairs, another guy had one arm, one man was amputated below both knees, while another competitor had one leg amputated below the knee. On the way to Canada we visited Disneyland and had a great time as we were escorted to the front of each ride and didn't have to queue.

We had been in America just one day when we visited the late millionaire Howard Hughes' amazing wooden plane, nicknamed the Spruce Goose. It was the largest plane ever to fly when Hughes lifted off from Long Beach, California on 2 November 1947. It is now at an aviation museum in McMinnville, Oregon, but it was still at Long Beach when I saw it. Still jetlagged, we did the hour-long tour of the Spruce Goose and we were a little bit early for our bus back to the hotel. So I wheeled out onto the beautifully manicured grounds, jumped out of my wheelchair, took off my hat and lay down and fell asleep under a palm tree.

I woke three-quarters of an hour later with $15 in my hat. I thought, 'Only in America, I love this place.'

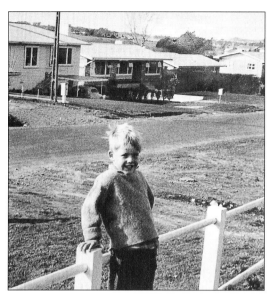

One of the few photos of me with legs, standing outside our house in Esk Street.

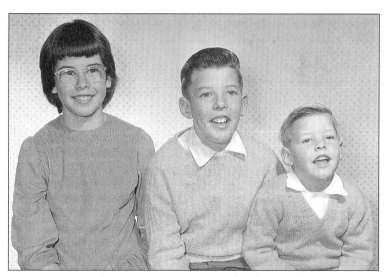

Family portrait time: sister Sue, brother Frank in the middle and me on the right.

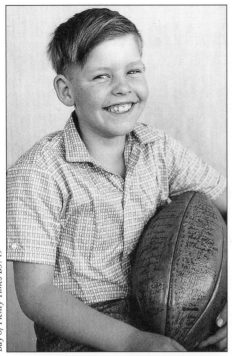

Public interest in my accident was quite high. The photo of me with one of my favourite nurses, Sister Wesselink, was taken by the Bay of Plenty Times, *and Colin Meads presented me with that wonderful rugby ball, signed by the 1959 All Blacks and Lions.*

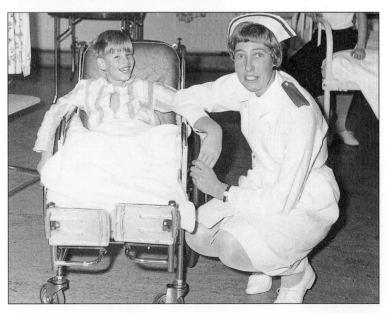

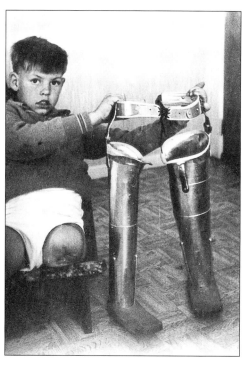

*The infamous rockers.
The belt secured the legs
to my body, and the
'foot' rocked to allow
me to 'walk'.*

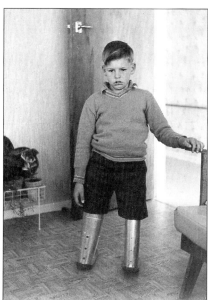

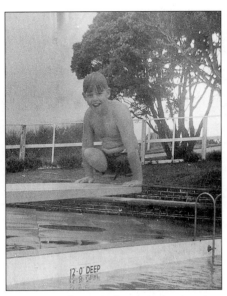

I was never keen on the idea of swimming when I had legs, but once Dave Franklin and Allan Guthrie got me enthused, there was no stopping me.

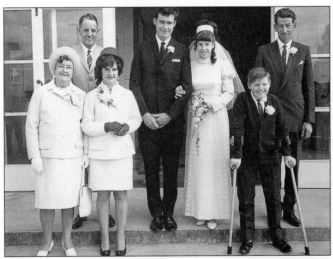

From left: my grandma Winifred, grandad Frank, Mum, my brother-in-law, Doug, my sister Sue, me and Dad at Sue's wedding.

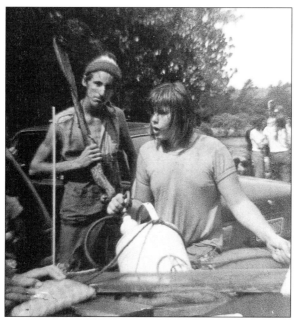

Having no legs certainly didn't stop me from having a good time. Top: Final preparations for the local raft race. Bottom: My lifeguard days. And see, it's harder than you think to stay balanced in a wheelchair.

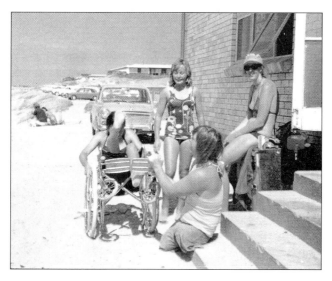

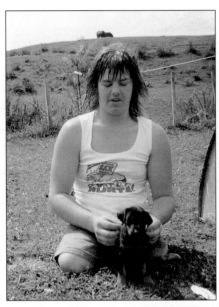

Astro, my sixteenth birthday present from Aunt Coral, was the runt of the litter and not expected to survive. But he did, and he became my constant companion.

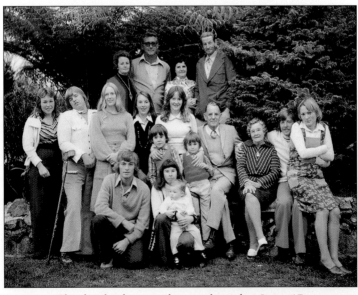

This family photograph was taken when I was 17.

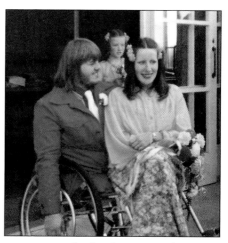

It's not every new bride who can justify sitting on her husband's lap for the wedding photos — but Elaine could. That's Nikki in the background.

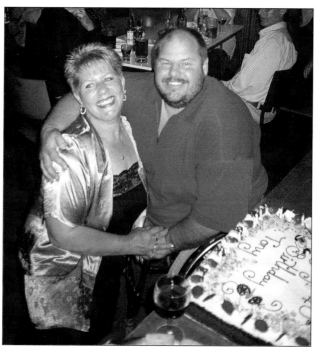

And all these years later, we're still very happy together.

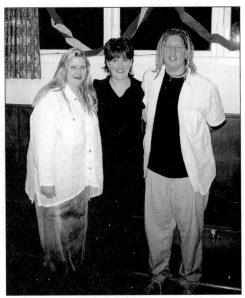

*Our wonderful kids: from left, Danie,
Nikki and Lucas.*

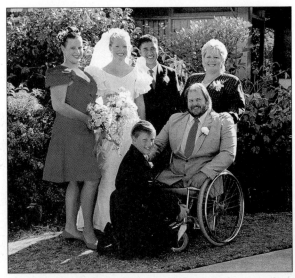

*The family gathers to welcome another member. Standing,
from left, Danie, Nikki and new husband Quentin, Elaine.
In front, Lucas and me.*

We also went to the huge department store, Sears Robuck, and team mate Steve Laing, who only had one arm, bought a small blow-up dinghy with oars. He met me outside the store and very proudly told me about his purchase. I stared at him in disbelief.

I said, 'Why did you buy that? You can't go anywhere except around in circles!'

He said, 'Oh, I didn't think about that.'

That was amazing — he had forgotten about his disability as he coped so well with his challenge. When we returned to New Zealand, we decided to give the blow-up dinghy a test run, so Steve and a couple of other guys from the team visited me in Tauranga. As we headed off in a car to a local river to launch the dinghy, my wife-to-be Elaine took a good look at us.

She said to us, 'I hope you don't get pulled over by the cops because they won't believe it, a guy with one arm and two guys with no legs — you're just bits and pieces!'

My next international competition was the 1982 FESPIC Games in Hong Kong and it took me a while to get used to the phenomenal heat and the 98 per cent humidity. I concentrated on basketball and we got through to the finals and won the silver. I also won gold in the discus, silver in the javelin and bronze in the shotput. One really annoying aspect of the competition was that the rules would be changed at every Games because the sport was developing, so we would be throwing different weights of equipment every time we competed. The senior men's discus in able-bodied competition weighs around 7 kilograms, but we threw a senior women's discus of around 5.5 kilograms. The javelin was the same — they upped us to senior women instead of junior men and there was a big difference because of the weight and the way they flew. Some were slimline and flew very well with a low trajectory, while others were a lot fatter and you needed to throw them higher in order for them to float further.

We found that, when sitting in a wheelchair, we could only throw about 30 metres as we couldn't gain the height needed for the javelins to reach their optimum potential. With the discus, it's the flat to the angle, the diameter of the discus and how it fits in the hand that makes it go further. I found it hard to grip the larger discus and throw it from the sitting position. A standing discus thrower rotates two or three times before letting it go, and also has the advantage of the force holding the discus into the palm of the hand. I could only swing two-thirds of a revolution, and that meant that often, in competition, the discus would fall out of my hand before I could throw it. But when I did let it go there was force behind it as I had big shoulders — this was an area of my body that I worked on building up.

Throughout my time representing New Zealand at the Games the weights were never the same at consecutive events. This was a hindrance as we would train with one weight and just before going to the Games the rules would change. Or we'd get to the Games and then the rule would change so we didn't have long to practice.

I stopped competing in athletics when I was in my late twenties because I was getting older and I had other commitments — my business, a young family, and my motor sports.

CHAPTER FOUR
WORK AND PLAY

*'Before I had the accident I could have done 10,000
things — been an All Black, played soccer at the
World Cup, been a world-class cyclist or a downhill
skier — but after the accident I could only do 8000
of those things.'*

I OVERHEARD Mum say to my sister once, 'You know, Tony's
going to be with us for the rest of our lives.' She really thought
that because of my disability I would always have to live with
her and Dad.

For a while I thought I would never have a girlfriend because people weren't going to accept me for who I was. But I
was determined that in this, like in other things in my life —
surf lifesaving, swimming — I wasn't going to be treated any
differently than my mates.

When I got my car I went out and did everything that young
guys my age did. I still had my great bunch of mates and I was
just a normal kid, I wasn't different and that acceptance was
important to me. It was the same thing with girls. I found
there were girls who would accept me for who I was, that
having no legs didn't matter. I had a lot more going for me and
did more things than some of the guys I hung out with. At 15,
I met my first girlfriend, Kay, who was a helper at athletics.
She taught me that there was someone out there for me, that I

could be loved and that people would accept me. Kay and I went around together for a couple of years, and I gained considerable personal confidence during this time. But I was single-minded about my sports activities and that meant we gradually drifted apart.

That first car was a Honda Civic automatic which was adapted so I could drive it. The hand control was like a motorbike throttle, as in you moved it around to accelerate, and then pulled it forwards to brake. There was also a separate cable for the hand control. There was only one problem when I picked up the car after it was adapted and took it for a spin for the first time — the accelerator was still connected and I didn't know it. When I got into the car, I still had my artificial legs on and my right leg accidentally rested on the accelerator.

My dad was in the car with me and we headed home along Tauranga's main road, Cameron Street. As we drove along the car's speed picked up; I pulled the hand control towards me to engage the brakes — but nothing happened.

By now Dad was becoming quite perturbed. He told me to slow down.

I told him I was trying to. The speed kept increasing, and I had to start weaving between cars as the speedo climbed past 50 kilometres an hour — the speed limit for the road. By now Dad was panicking, and this usually mild-mannered man was yelling at me to stop. I yelled back that I was *trying* to — I was yanking the brake as far forward as possible without breaking it. Still the car went faster. I looked ahead and saw we were coming to a major intersection and I knew that if we didn't stop we'd have a serious accident. Luckily Dad had the presence of mind to tell me to turn off the ignition key and cut the engine. I did that, the engine stopped and we coasted to the side of the road, just before the intersection.

When Dad and I calmed down we tried to work out what

was wrong with the car — apart from it being possessed. Then I looked down and saw where my right foot was resting. After that incident, I've always had the accelerator cable disconnected in all my cars, even though I wasn't wearing my artificial legs when I was older.

When I was a teen, the car gave me so much more independence — I could get to athletics by myself and get out and be a normal guy. But I think my independence was hard on my mum and dad as, after years of devoting so much time to me, I didn't rely on them any more. They, of course, deny that and say they were relieved when I could drive myself around. My parents did worry when I drove by myself, especially on long trips. They had heard about a disabled driver who was targeted by some hoons because they saw his wheelchair on the back of the car. But once I got my dog Astro, my parents felt he'd protect me if I got into that kind of trouble. Astro was a Doberman pup and was my sixteenth birthday present from my Aunty Coral, Mum's sister. He was the runt of the litter and wasn't expected to live, so they couldn't sell him with the other pedigree pups — but he soon grew into a large dog who went everywhere with me, even to school, usually on the back seat of my car. I'd fold down the back seat and put a mattress in for him; with him in the car and the windows open, nobody would dare go near. At morning tea, lunchtime and school breaks I'd let him out for a run.

I also worried my parents when I said I was going out for a drive for an hour — then came back home at 4 a.m. because I had been fishing at the wharf.

I felt those worries were the same for most parents of teenagers. I respected my mum and dad, and always made sure I came home after a night out with the boys. I was also always bringing my mates home to swim in the pool. My parents were really good about that — they always preferred that I brought my mates home to stay overnight if I needed to. And, of course, like other guys my age we thought we were men when it came to alcohol, although it didn't play a big part in our lives. Once Dad let us have a drink of his home-brew beer and after half a jug I ended up on my back on our front lawn — talk about being legless!

While I wasn't into boozing, I was a hoon in my car. I did wheelies in supermarket car parks after hours or I'd find a paddock somewhere and zoom around in it. I had the latest Honda Civic while my mates had Morris Minor 1000s and Minis and I had the quickest car, especially when it came to drag racing. It got to the point where I was 'the man' because I had the nicest car.

I'd often drive to Auckland to visit a friend I made through the disabled games — Trevor Cullen. Sometimes mates from Tauranga would tag along too, usually Porky McGill and Brian Hartley. When we were in Auckland we'd go to the Saturday night speedway at Western Springs then on the way home on Sunday we'd go to the drag racing at Meremere.

This boosted my interest in motor sport even more. But that was a part of my life that was still to come. Before I got seriously interested in motor racing, I got a job.

I had artistic talent but I was never very academic. I didn't really enjoy my last years in school, probably because so much more was happening in my life — I had been around the world by the time I was 16 because of the Paralympics. So I left school at 16 with School Certificate in art, English and maths. I got 18 per cent for geography — hey, I might not have been able to find those countries on a map, but I'd probably been to them!

When I left school Mum told me I had to get a job like 'normal' people. There was no sitting around sponging off my parents. But I went through a period where I thought, 'I don't have any legs, what am I going to do?' At one stage I thought that no one could blame me for not doing anything — I had no legs, so who'd want to hire me? I soon snapped out of that. I always knew I'd make something out of my life, not be a bum sitting around all day on my bum.

While I was at school I worked part-time doing signwriting jobs on stockcars and making a few posters in the basement at Mum and Dad's place. To do the writing on the cars, I'd either sit on the floor or, to get me to the right height, I'd sit on a beer crate. The people next door had a shop so I wrote price tickets for them, and that led to a part-time job at the nearby Woolworths store. While my mates were earning $10 a week on a paper run I was making $50, $80 to $100 doing signwriting. That led to my decision to become a signwriter — I knew I had a talent, and it was going to earn me some money.

My first job was ticket writing for Woolworths full time. This entailed writing prices on cards — say, for toasters on sale. The tickets all had to be written by hand with felt tips and marker pens. I was sent to Auckland to do courses, and I became very good at ticket writing. People made careers out of that in those days, but it wasn't earning me enough money. So after eight months I applied for a job as a ticket writer for the New World chain of supermarkets. The vacancy was for a new store in Tauranga, but the interview was in Whakatane with Allan Able, the owner of the store, and Eddie Peden, the store manager. I showed them my credentials and some of my work and they took me on. This was great for me because I always felt that the Woolworths position was a little bit of a sympathy job — give the poor disabled guy a job — but Allan and Eddie hired me on my merits. There I was, aged 17, on a wage, in my own office based with the administration staff in the upstairs loft area of the Tauranga supermarket. I had a list of work I had to do but basically I was in charge of all the ticket writing in the supermarket and anything I wanted I could have — paints, pens and so on. It was great experience for me and it gave me confidence because I was treated as an equal, although I still had to wear my legs because the bosses wanted that image, me looking 'normal' — it was a bit of a stipulation.

But, after a year, I decided to move on. I wanted to get into signwriting, not just writing price cards. I had been doing part-time signwriting for the Tauranga Museum — restoring old signs, creating new ones — so I was approached to work there full time.

At this time I had stopped wearing my artificial legs altogether; for work, I could easily climb up the scaffolding (as I do now in my seminars). Those years of climbing trees as a kid really paid off. I've never gone back to wearing the legs.

Unfortunately, there wasn't much call for a signwriter in a wheelchair in Tauranga in those days so I never had an apprenticeship as a signwriter. It was not from want of trying — I had approached all the signwriting companies in Tauranga ten times over asking for a job and had been turned down for the same reasons. They'd say to me, 'You can't climb ladders, you can't drive a truck, so you're no good to us.' I was disheartened at that as I knew I had the ability to be a signwriter — I just needed someone to give me a chance. But I was motivated and I wanted to learn, so before I took up the job at the museum I went out and found myself some work experience as a signwriter.

A friend's brother, Trevor Moss, had a signwriting business in nearby Hamilton, so I worked for him for three months. It was a fantastic experience, learning the business first-hand and gaining invaluable knowledge about signwriting. As a result, I started work at the museum with important skills that enabled me to work professionally as a signwriter. The museum job was supposed to be for six months, but eighteen months later I was still there and I wasn't complaining. The job taught me so many new skills. I learned to become creative. I would recreate the old flowery-style signs and search through old books to discover the way signs were painted years before.

I had a great time working at the museum. I'm one of those people who enjoy doing the things they're passionate about, and are eager to develop their skills in these activities. I am still like that — learning how to improve my skills, be it signwriting or speech-making. There's no point plodding along at the same old job, not learning anything or improving yourself. That's a waste of your time and your energy, you're just going backwards. Get out there and make some challenges for yourself — no matter how big or small.

And that's what happened to me at the museum. Sure, I could have just plodded along, I was doing what I always wanted to do — signwriting — and it was enjoyable work, but I knew I wanted to do more than that in my life. I met a young guy, Jim Muir, who was working at the museum doing screenprinting. We became friends and soon decided to start our own signwriting and screenprinting business, Printed Images and Signs.

Jim lived in a block of units near the museum with his wife and young kids and didn't have a car, so I would often drive him home. One day he pointed out his neighbour, Elaine, a young divorcée with a little girl, five-year-old Nikki.

I expressed my interest in her but was quickly put in my place by Jim.

'Forget about her, you can't afford her,' were Jim's immortal words to me. Little did I realise that it wouldn't be too long before I would be married to Elaine, and, as she jokes over twenty years later, I still can't afford her!

But in the museum days I was 19, ambitious and confident. Jim and I began working out of the large basement of Elaine's unit and we went around town touting for work and

I proved to be a handy marketing man, pushing to get jobs for our business. I used some of the money from the trust fund to start the business and buy resources for screenprinting T-shirts and painting signs. Business was fine for a while — we got plenty of signwriting work, but not much screenprinting. Unfortunately, Jim couldn't signwrite, while I could also screenprint; so, eventually I bought Jim out and took the business over completely.

While I was doing well working for myself I was also asked if I'd take some night school classes in ticket writing at the local polytechnic. It was an eight-week course held one night a week. The money was good, and I enjoyed passing on my skills to other people.

One of the guys in my night school class, Des Robertson, was working as an apprentice at a large signwriting business in Tauranga, called Commercial Signs. One night Des told me that his boss was looking for a new worker and I should apply. Working for myself was okay, but it was a bit of a struggle too; I didn't always have money, so I thought I needed to get a proper job.

Lance Styles was managing Commercials Signs at that time and he was hesitant to hire me. He looked at me, frowning, and gave me the usual excuses about why I couldn't do the job — 'You can't climb ladders, you can't drive a truck, you're no use to me.'

But I was determined to work as a signwriter and I now had experience behind me. So I said to him, 'Give me a chance, you won't be sorry, I can do all of that stuff.' He said he had other applicants for the job and would get back to me. Fortunately for me Lance didn't like the other applicants so he gave me a chance. I was given three months to prove myself and at the end of that time I approached Lance and asked him what he thought of my work. I need not have worried — Lance was so impressed he made me foreman.

Later on I found out that Commercial Signs' owner, Alan Wright, was against Lance hiring me. At that time, Commercial Signs was both a signwriting and screenprinting business but in 1986 Alan split them up and sold the signwriting side to Lance and his wife Kathy, and the screenprinting to Ray Herdman, a former pig farmer. Lance ran the signwriting side while Kathy kept the books and was in charge of the office.

I joined Commercials Signs when I was 20, working with five other blokes as a signwriter. They became my mates. We'd have a beer after work, they'd invite me to social events and we'd do things together at the weekends. At last I was doing what I wanted to do — professional signwriting — but I still had my goals. There were so many other things in my life that I wanted to achieve.

I've often found that the people I worked with seemed to have goals that were lower than mine; most of them settled for mediocrity whereas I was trying to strive for a little bit more. Not only did I want to be a professional signwriter, I also wanted my own business, and I wanted to achieve so much more in my life. When I die I want people to remember who I am and what I've achieved. We're only around for such a short time so why shouldn't we try to strive to do so much in that time — set goals, try your hardest to achieve them? It's not much to ask, is it?

Sure, I had a setback when I was nine. But that didn't stop me getting out there and trying my hardest to make a difference. As I've always said, before I had the accident I could have done 10,000 things — been an All Black, played soccer at the World Cup, been a world-class cyclist or a downhill skier — but after the accident I could only do 8000 of those things. And that's the way we should look at life — it's full of opportunities.

I was happy working for Lance and Kathy for a few years, but when they acrimoniously split I left Commercial Signs as I didn't like the atmosphere there — life is too short to deal with such tension at work.

CHAPTER FIVE
DADDY NO LEGS

*'Why should the world label me disabled when I have
done more in my life than most people will ever
dream of? — and I haven't finished yet! Why do we
need to categorise people?'*

As MY business life excelled, so too did my private life, after
my initial self-doubts about ever having a relationship. I became pretty confident after a few girlfriends; Elaine was the
hardest to impress.

I used to see her walking and I'd offer her a lift in my car
but she always said no. As she tells it, she was walking for
exercise and rejected the offers as she was trying to keep fit. I
had one of the flashest cars among my mates, as I'd traded in
the Civic for a red Datsun 120Y. But Elaine thought I was a
big head and that I acted like 'Jack the Lad' in the car. And
there I was thinking I was pretty cool. That's women for you!

Elaine says in those days I acted very confidently in my car
because people couldn't tell that I didn't have legs and they
wouldn't have believed that a 'disabled' person could drive
such a car. Again, it's all perception.

But despite her rejection of my gallant offers of a lift, I
slowly began to win her over, thanks to an episode down at
the local pub.

I was drinking with a big group of my friends one night

when I saw Elaine enter the pub. I called her over and did the 'disabled' line on her that I had found most successful in the past. I asked her if she would go up to the bar and buy me a drink as it was too awkward for me to get to the crowded bar in my wheelchair. And while she's up there she should get herself a drink too. Elaine fell for it, no problem. Well, actually, she knew it was a pick up line but it was a good excuse to get some free drinks. As she saw it, I was sitting with a big group of mates and they could have easily got my drinks for me. But she came back with the drinks and sat with me. All evening Elaine went up to the bar and got the drinks for us, and we chatted. At the end of the night I offered her a ride home and this time she accepted.

When we got to the car I opened the passenger door for her and she got in. I then went to the boot, put my chair in there and then shuffled to the driver's side. As I hopped into the car Elaine was mortified. There she was, sitting in the car like Lady Muck while I'd had to put my wheelchair in by myself. She felt awful that she didn't offer to help me. Not that I minded; she was treating me like a 'normal' date and as she later explained, 'It never entered my head that Tony would need help as he seemed so able and acted if he could take care of himself.'

Soon I began to spend a lot of time around at Elaine's house with her and Nikki.

Elaine was originally from England and moved to Tauranga with her parents when she was a teenager. Her parents lived nearby and Elaine had been on her own for a while, bringing up Nikki as well as working.

Elaine had explained to Nikki that I had no legs and the first time I went to Elaine's house Nikki was all revved up to answer the door. But when I knocked on the door, Nikki chickened out and told her mum to get the door. She was soon relaxed with me and we got on great, and so did Elaine and me. We had the same sense of humour and, as she was eight years older than I was, I appreciated her maturity. Also, Elaine never treated me any differently from anyone else and couldn't care less that I didn't have any legs.

She was also attracted to my movie star good looks, winning personality and charm, of course. Okay, Elaine liked the fact I was so outgoing and fun-loving, and that's what she needed coming out of a bad marriage.

I paid a lot of attention to her — she says she couldn't get rid of me — and I started spending nights at her house — much to my mum's displeasure. Mum had misgivings because Elaine was older than me and had a child. On our wedding day she even made Elaine promise that she'd love me forever, and she reminds Elaine of that often. Elaine's reply is, 'Yeah I probably will, but that doesn't mean I have to live with him forever.' Charming.

Elaine's mum, Eileen, wasn't happy when she heard her daughter was going out with me. She thought that I wasn't going to be a provider because I had no legs, but Elaine's dad, Reg Sumsion, didn't mind. As he saw it, I had a job at the time so why wouldn't I have a job forever?

Our relationship wasn't accepted by everyone, though. Elaine's best friend, Trish Bermingham, was very shocked. She came around for lunch at Elaine's unit when Elaine and I first got together. I was sitting at the table and everything was fine until I jumped down off my chair and onto my bum. Trish got a bit of a fright and Elaine didn't see Trish for two weeks. But Elaine is very self-confident, and when she makes up her mind it usually stays that way; so she made Trish see all the good things about me. Trish had been through the hard times of Elaine's first marriage, so Elaine made Trish realise how different I was from her ex-husband, and how totally right I was for Elaine.

But Elaine herself had a misgiving or two at the beginning. One night when we first started going out I had fallen asleep on the couch while Elaine was watching television. She looked at me and realised how small I was, just over three feet. She thought to herself, 'I'm really going out with a man with no legs! So what, is there anything wrong with that? No, because you're not going out with what's on the outside, it's what's on the inside that counts and that's completely different.'

She's a wise woman. If only more people thought like that.

Elaine's seen me with my artificial legs on only once. She came around to Mum and Dad's house soon after we started dating and I went into my bedroom and struggled into my legs — I hadn't worn them for a few years. I thumped down the corridor in them and flung open the living room door and stood there, very proud of myself. Elaine took one look at me and said, 'Get them off, you look ridiculous.'

By the time Jim and I started running the screenprinting and signwriting business from the basement, Elaine and I were living together.

Danielle Christiansen was born by Caesarean section at Tauranga Hospital on 1 March 1979. It was a fantastic day; I remember clearly the nurses bringing Danie (as she's always known) to me while Elaine was still in theatre. I couldn't believe this tiny creature was really my daughter. I checked to see she had both legs then I weighed her, bathed her and spent three and a half hours with my newborn daughter. Unfortunately, new mum Elaine wasn't impressed that I wasn't around when she came out of theatre. I was in big trouble.

There was one memorable occasion when Danie was a baby and Elaine had to go to my parents' home to pick up something. I was left in charge of eight-year-old Nikki and tiny Danie, who was asleep at the time. No problems, I thought.

What problems could a baby cause? I'd saved lives and

won gold medals. So caring for a baby — and her big sister — would be sweatless. Besides, it was only for half an hour; Danie couldn't possibly cause any trouble in that time.

Oh, how young and naïve I was.

Danie woke up unexpectedly and started screaming and I couldn't placate her. I tried every trick in the book but there was a problem — I couldn't carry her around to try to soothe her as I needed my arms to shuffle around on. Nikki couldn't cope with the noise — and I wasn't too happy either. There was only one thing to do — admit defeat.

Elaine had barely arrived at my mum's place when I made the frantic call for her to come home — immediately — if not sooner. After that, Elaine didn't leave me alone with Danie again while she was tiny.

Although I had Danie, I always treated Nikki as a daughter and she regarded me, and still does, as her dad. I hate the word 'step' — as in stepdaughter. It annoys me when people say I'm Nikki's stepdad. I'm whatever she wants me to be. She has no contact with her natural father, but it wouldn't worry me if she did because we have such a strong relationship. Once you call someone 'step', it labels them. One of the things I feel strongly about is this need we have to label people; we do it because it makes *us* feel comfortable.

They label me disabled.

Why should the world label me disabled when I have done more in my life than most people will ever dream of? — and I haven't finished yet! Why do we need to categorise people?

But labels and people's perceptions didn't stop Elaine and me. We sold Elaine's place and while we were building our new house at Welcome Bay, just outside of Tauranga, we got married. I had decided earlier that year that Elaine and I would marry — I just needed to convince her. After her first marriage she was reluctant to get hitched again, but I was persistent and convinced her it was the right thing to do. We got married on 23 October 1980, four days after my 21st birthday.

I had moved my signwriting business to a big shed at our Welcome Bay home and was teaching night classes. We also had the two girls and Elaine and I decided we didn't want any more children. So we went to see Dr Mountford about me getting the snip. At first he was reluctant because I was just 23, but I was adamant so he agreed to go ahead. As he said to me, 'I seem to be always cutting things off you, Tony.'

Six weeks after the vasectomy I came home from a racing weekend away and Elaine told me she had news for me — she was five months pregnant!

She had been having problems with the contraceptive pill, hence the snip, but had been feeling unwell for a few months. So while I was away motor racing she went to see her doctor who quickly diagnosed the problem — she was expecting. She went to tell my mum, who knew about the vasectomy, and my mum said, 'Who's the father?'

Mother-and-daughter-in-law relations were strained for a while after that.

On 14 August 1982, Lucas Jon Christiansen was born and this time it was a normal delivery and I watched him being born. It was a truly amazing experience for me and one I will never forget.

Once Danie and Lucas could crawl and then walk, I'd spend a lot of time on the floor with them, rolling about. When they became toddlers they loved playing with me as I was their height.

The kids were pretty oblivious to the fact their daddy didn't have any legs — I was never regarded by them as being out of the ordinary and they became quite blasé about me. They just accepted me and even joked about me. Danie used to call me Daddy No Legs or Neil — as in the joke: What do you call a man with no legs? Neil.

The kids even used to buy me socks for Christmas. Cheeky all right, but that's what I'm like. I'm not sensitive about not having any legs and I often joke about it — hey, you've got to get on with life, not sit around and feel sorry for yourself, you're not going to get ahead that way.

My kids' nonchalance became obvious when they started bringing friends home. Elaine and I would have to remind them to tell their little pals that 'daddy has no legs' and it was obvious when they forgot because the moment the kids clapped eyes on me their mouths would drop and they'd stare at me. When Lucas started school he had problems convincing his class about me during morning talks. He'd come home with some mates, point at me and say, 'See, I told you he didn't have any legs.' We'd go to school events and the kids would forget to let people know that I was in a wheelchair, and a lot of the kids would stare at me.

We were just like any other family, though. For eight years we'd go away during the Christmas holidays to nearby Lake Rotoiti with friends and their kids. I'd join in with all the activities like cricket, and we'd take our speedboat along too. We had some laughs during those lake holidays and one incident stands out for me. We were on the lake with our speedboat when a warden came up to us and told us we weren't supposed to be there.

He asked me to step out of the boat.

I said, 'No I can't.'

The warden said, 'I said, can you please step out of the boat.'

I said, 'No, I can't, I can hop if you like, but I can't step out.'

The warden said, 'What do you mean?'

So I hopped out of the boat and the warden nearly fell off the pier.

As I got more into my motor racing our summers were spent at the track instead of the lake. Elaine wasn't into the racing but the two girls were; actually, Nikki was really there for the boys. She'd disappear when we arrived at the track and turn up at the end of the races, but Danie would stick around, though it wasn't too long before she went off too.

The kids found that there was a bonus to having a dad with no legs. Lucas used to say it was great because I was the only dad who could play in McDonald's playground because Ronald said you had to be under four feet tall!

One family holiday we went to Disneyland and I wasn't allowed on a ride because I was too short. The measurement was supposed to be from your bum to your head as you were strapped into the ride and I had a big enough torso to stay in the ride. But when I tried to join the kids on the ride, the operator told me I couldn't go on because I was too short. I complained to management and they later let me on the ride. The problem with some of those places in America is they are terrified of being sued. But the bonus of being in a wheelchair at Disneyland was that my family and I didn't have to queue for rides — we'd be sent up the exit and straight on to the ride. Then, when we finished the ride, the operator would ask if we wanted to go again.

These days, if I'm at a theme park in America, I always go to the main office first and tell them that, given all my achievements, it's fine for me to go on the rides. So they ring up the rides that I want to go to in advance and tell them that I'm coming. It's so embarrassing to turn up to a ride and not be allowed to go on it while the operator checks with his manager to see if I can. It's not worth the hassle.

No matter where we are holidaying, though, we meet people who know me. It's happened in America, in Australia, at airports, beaches, everywhere. Elaine reckons I can't go anywhere without bumping into someone I know — be it someone from Tauranga or a person who has been to one of my speeches. It never ceases to amaze Elaine that so many people know me — it must be my face that people remember!

While I was active in my sports, I also got involved in activities with my kids. Lucas played soccer when he was at primary school. I was assistant to the assistant coach, and I always went to watch Lucas play. But one day I took him to soccer and no coaches turned up, so it became my job. All the kids stood around and I was telling them how to play when one of the kids said to me, 'You don't have any legs, what would you know?' So I got out of my wheelchair and sat in front of the mini goal, and said, 'The first kid that gets the ball past me gets an ice cream.' And they kicked balls from every direction, but they never got one past me. From that day their attitude towards me changed — I was Lucas's dad or Mr C and I could do ordinary things with them. I just had to show them.

At Tauranga Boys High School Lucas played basketball when he was 14 and 15, and I coached the team since I played wheelchair basketball. When they started playing, his team had watched too much of the American basketball stars Michael Jordan and Shaquille O'Neal. So they were doing all these flowery moves when shooting, but the opposition took the ball away from them. Through showing them moves, I soon got them back to basics and they won the tournament they played in. I used to join in their practice too, although I have to admit I cheated when I was playing one-on-one. Although I was pretty fast in the wheelchair the boys could outrun me, but sometimes I'd spin around in the chair and run over their feet! From then on they'd go right around me and give me more room.

These days, my kids say I have to win at any cost. Elaine

looks at my attitude this way: 'His motivation is that he likes to win. If you train to be the best, you can be. Tony wants to win, to be the best.' I have to agree with her. Being involved in sport and participating is important, but I want to do the best that I can and winning is the best. People remember who took the gold medal, they don't remember who came second or third.

I also set goals and this is one of the most important reasons that I've done so well in business, sports and at home. Although none of my kids are seriously into sport, I think they each set their own goals in their life.

Nikki has Elaine's cooking talents and works part-time as a gateau decorator. She married Quentin Jacob six years ago, then travelled overseas and lived in Britain for a while. In 1997 they had a son, Houston, and now I play with the lad like I did when my kids were little.

Lucas has a goal to be a chef and has finished an introduction to hospitality course at the local technical institute.

Since Danie left school she's been working as a Christian youth coordinator locally, organising venues for Christian bands to play in the area and arranging billets for them. She is also a talented singer and her goal is to travel with a Christian youth band.

Danie has trouble with my 'fame' in Tauranga and is always referred to as Tony Christiansen's daughter — she hates it. She wants everyone to know she's Danie, not just someone's daughter and I think that's what makes her so outgoing and forward. I also think Danie's learnt to be outgoing from me, and she listens to what I talk about in my speeches. For example, Danie began babysitting this year and I asked her if she told the family how much she was going to charge. She hadn't. I said, 'Why not? What if they only give you ten dollars for your six hours of child minding? The expectation is that when you're babysitting during the day it's ten dollars an hour and five dollars at night when the kids are asleep. That's what's going to happen to you — people are always going to give you less than what you require. So you tell them from the start what your expectations are.'

So she took this lesson on board — and the next day came to me to ask for a loan for a car that she had fallen in love with! She told me what her expectations were, how she intended to pay me back the money — the works. She had it all planned, and even back-up arguments if I said no straight away. Although I admired her effort, and the fact that she had paid attention to my advice, she didn't get the loan — and she's still driving her old car. Besides, the owner was asking too much for the car.

Actually, there was something in the car story that reflects Danie's attitude to my 'fame' in Tauranga. When she rang the owner to ask for a test drive she asked him if he could bring the car to our house as her dad wanted to have a look. The owner said no, she'd have to come to him and bring her dad with him.

'I can't,' said Danie, 'my dad's in a wheelchair . . .'

And before she could finish her sentence the owner asked, 'Is your dad Tony Christiansen?'

Danie wasn't impressed. She was just trying to be a prospective car buyer, not race car driver Tony Christiansen's daughter.

Elaine reckons I have high expectations for the kids, although I know they have a tough path to follow with me as a role model. Some people expect my kids and Elaine to be like me, very motivated and goal-oriented, but they are different from me. Sure, sometimes it upsets me that the kids aren't as motivated as I am. For example, Lucas hasn't gone for his driver's licence, although he talks about buying an old car and restoring it. I'd love to help him with that goal, but I'd like to see him start working towards it before I lend a hand. A self-improvement course taught me to value my family and children and be thankful for what they are and not what they aren't. I learned that the children are different from me, and I appreciate they are their own people.

Elaine worked for many years as a chef but a bad back injury put paid to that and she is still in constant pain from it. She loves decorating our homes and helped design our latest one. In the new house there has been some compensation made for me — the house is mostly carpeted as I'm on my bum all the time. The wheelchair stays in the garage as it's easier for me to get around without it, although the doors are very wide in case I need to bring the wheelchair in. We have a sliding shower in our *en suite*, and the light switches have been lowered for me. Apart from stairs up to Danie and Lucas's bedrooms and living space, there are no steps in the house. The kitchen benches are normal size as I can't cook (and with so many chefs in the house there's no need for me to) but although I can take care of myself, I'm not much help around the house for Elaine.

It annoys Elaine that in restaurants the staff talk to her rather than me and, when we reach our table, they always take my chair away and expect me to sit at the table in my wheelchair, whereas I prefer to sit on the chair. To add insult to injury, the waiters always ask Elaine what I'd like to eat, not me directly. They'd only need to spend a second with me to realise I have all my faculties and am very capable of talking — hey, I do it for a living.

It's all about perception.

When Elaine and I go to dances we don't sit on the side watching, we get out on the dance floor and have a jive, with me dancing in my wheelchair. And just about every time we've done that I'm inundated with old, grey-haired ladies rushing across the room to ask me to dance.

Is it my handsome looks and charming personality that attract them? Elaine has another theory. She says that the old ladies don't rush to ask any other males in the room to dance, and that they only ask me because they think it's their good deed for the day — be nice to the man in the wheelchair. I think that's unfair — it must be my aftershave that attracts them.

When Elaine married me she didn't realise how much she was going to have to do by herself. I can't bring the shopping in from the car and when the kids were little I couldn't carry them from the car when they were asleep. When she first met me it didn't occur to her that she'd be left to do all these things herself, as I was so active. She says she's had to take on half my responsibilities. Elaine's joke to her friends is that she was going to go to the social welfare and ask to go on the benefit. They'd say, 'How can you, you're married?'

She'd say, 'I've only got half a husband so I should get half a benefit.'

But Elaine doesn't have to do anything personally for me — I'm quite capable of taking care of myself. And I'm not totally useless around the house — I do my share, too. I mow the lawns on my ride-on mower and it's great practice for speedway.

When we are away from home, Elaine usually takes care of our travel arrangements, especially when we are at an airport. She books us in and checks in the luggage and arranges for us to be escorted onto the plane ahead of the other passengers. There's only one problem when we travel overseas — Elaine hates flying, so much so that she has to take a pill to calm her down. One trip she took the pill before we boarded so she was feeling very 'happy' when the flight attendant approached us in the departure lounge and said she'd escort us onto the plane. The flight attendant led the way, with me following and Elaine behind me. As we came to the gate, Elaine thought she'd take a short cut past some passengers and meet us at the entrance. Unfortunately, she was too zonked to take in her surroundings and walked face first into a huge window instead. Poor thing nearly knocked herself out and she had to be helped on the plane instead of me for a change. I didn't let her live that down for months.

When I fly alone I try to travel with just hand luggage that I can carry on my lap in the wheelchair instead of attempting to check in suitcases. I still find that airport staff take one look at me in a wheelchair and think I'm mentally challenged. I feel like saying, 'Hello, just because I'm in a wheelchair doesn't mean I can't do things. Hey, I can even fly a plane.'

When I get on board and am in my seat one of the flight crew takes the wheelchair and stores it in the hold. I move around the aircraft on my bum and, once the plane lands, the flight attendants bring the wheelchair to me. Most airlines are fantastic, and they make sure there is someone to help me when we land. But Brisbane airport is terrible — the ground crew won't get anything from the hold, so my wheelchair must go through to baggage claim. Consequently I have to use one of the airport's wheelchairs, and they are usually old. It's like wearing someone else's shoes. I hope the ground crew don't read this or I'll never see my wheelchair again when I next fly to Brisbane.

Elaine found a family tradition of mine from when I lived at home very strange. On the anniversary of my accident, Mum would cook a chicken, which was a treat for us from our usual fare of mince and sausages. But Elaine joked that the reason we had a chicken was so that I could get the legs. Cheeky!

My mum calls me arrogant, because I am so dogged in my determination to succeed. She sometimes wonders where I get my motivation from. Was I born with it? Was it because of the accident? Was it due to the people who helped me when I was young — Grandad, swimming coaches Allan Guthrie and Dave Franklin, athletic coaches Peter Pollock and Doug Moore? Or was it due to my parents' encouragement? I think it is a result of all of those factors.

As Mum says, I was always a handful — well, I like to think that I was just enthusiastic as a child — so I was always going to do something with my life. The challenge of having no legs just made me more determined to succeed. Although I am a positive person I do have my 'down' moments — like most people. I don't look at having no legs as a handicap, but sometimes I get despondent and it's usually the little things that trigger it — like going into the kitchen and not being able to reach something on the shelves. I think, 'Bugger, if only I had legs then I'd be able to reach that!' but then the moment passes. I also get frustrated at times because there are certain things I want to achieve and I have no one to turn to to get advice from. I don't know many people like me so I try my best to muddle along until I find a way of achieving my goal.

People also tell me I'm lucky — I've got a healthy family, a loving wife, beautiful home, great job and I've been successful in many, many aspects of my life. But I disagree. Luck is winning Lotto. I'm fortunate.

I'm fortunate that I've been able to get out and do so many things in my life instead of sitting at home moping. I'm fortunate that my kids are healthy and smart and just fantastic people. I'm fortunate that I met Elaine and that we've been married for over twenty years now.

But I've also worked very hard to achieve things in my life.

When I was younger and was rejected by signwriting companies in Tauranga, I didn't give up my goal and sit around feeling sorry for myself. I was determined to become a signwriter. Sure, I was fortunate that Lance from Commercial

Signs saw my potential and took me on, but then I worked very hard to show everyone that I could do the job. In my speaking career I was fortunate that a few people saw I had a talent for public speaking, but it was up to me to push myself into it.

And that's what life is all about. Don't sit there waiting for your goal or life-long ambition to come knocking on your door. Go out there and grab it. Don't expect promotion or recognition unless you're willing to put in the hard work to achieve it. You've got to do it all yourself, push yourself and if you truly want it, your goal will be achieved.

CHAPTER SIX

THE SKY'S THE LIMIT

*'I achieved another goal and it taught me that you
should take every opportunity that is offered.'*

WHILE I was surf lifesaving I gave up go-kart racing, but I went
back to it when I was 26. This time I entered a higher level and
became quite good, racing competitively around the North
Island.

During that time I had an interest in speedway and was at
Tauranga's Baypark race track doing the time keeping. A couple of mates of mine had midget cars and I realised that because
of the simple mechanisms of the cars — accelerator, brake and
one gear — this was a sport for me. So I started to look around
and eventually I found a midget car with an old Bedford engine that a guy had sitting in his shed. I bought it for $4,000
while Elaine was in England visiting her relatives. She wasn't
impressed when I rang her up to tell her. 'How's the trip? How
are things? Guess what, I've bought a midget car.' It was easier
to break it to her when she was 10,000 miles away.

I had a mechanical background thanks to my dad and the
time we'd spent tinkering around with the go-kart. When I
was 16, I built a T-bucket hotrod for a school project in engineering class. I built the chassis at school and took it home to
finish it. Although I have a talent with engines I didn't want
to become a mechanic when I left school because it seemed

impractical for me. I couldn't see myself leaning over car bonnets. In fact, I wanted to be a precision engineer, but again, it seemed like a lot of lugging stuff around and carrying things from one point to another. And I suppose I got talked out of it by people, it wasn't a very practical career for me. I'm sure I would have been very good at it though.

I raced the midget at Baypark in the open class and did really well, and I also won the championships at Western Springs and Meremere.

Those years of go-kart racing had taught me driving skills, and hooning around in my Honda Civic had taught me a trick or two as well. Also, I was competitive and determined, I wasn't a hothead who raced on the track for the fun of it. Instead, I combined the skills I learnt from athletics and surf lifesaving competitions in order to formulate strategies. I had that 'no fear' attitude that let me take risks other drivers may not have done.

It was a great social time for me and I had a good bunch of mates. They nicknamed my cars 'Tonails' and called me after the Star Wars character R2D2, because I looked like him with my racing suit and helmet on as I shuffled along on my bum.

I adapted the midget car slightly using hand controls with a twist grip and brake, but I had to steer it with one hand. So to help I added power steering and was one of the first guys to do so. It made steering so much easier for me and it worked really well. Then I progressed onto another midget, a later model Holbar with a Volkswagen engine, which was the good gear at the time and I did extremely well. Then I had quite a heavy crash at Kihikihi a few years ago.

It was the last race of the last meeting of the season and it was just one of those things that happens — fate, you could call it. It was late in the afternoon, and the track was really dusty, I came around a corner and a guy had spun out in front of me. I hit him square on; my car climbed up over him and it went one or two metres in the air. It barrel-rolled three or four times and as it came down it fell apart. I wasn't hurt, just pretty shaken, and the incident certainly knocked my confidence. I decided I didn't want to race in the midget class any more.

But, of course, you should never say never.

I'd previously had a bad accident when racing at Baypark while my sister Sue and my kids were watching. I hit the wall and was taken to hospital with suspected concussion.

Elaine had just finished working at the restaurant and was having a shower when Sue and the kids turned up. The first thing they said to her was, 'He's okay' so Elaine knew immediately that I had been in an accident.

'Tony's at the hospital and he's hit the wall but he's okay,' Sue said.

Meanwhile, at the hospital, I was causing dramas. I had my racing suit cut off and I was just in my undies, with a blanket over me, when they carried me into the emergency department on a stretcher. I was lying in the middle of the stretcher to even out the weight because there had been a mishap earlier at the track. When the ambulance crew put me onto the stretcher there I was positioned at one end, so when they lifted the stretcher I slid off it head first and landed back on the ground.

Not a good start.

When I arrived at the hospital the doctors came in and looked at my legless form and said, 'Oh my God, what happened?' When they lifted up the blanket they realised I was an amputee so they started examining my stumps, asking how I lost my legs, who did the operation and saying what a good job Dr Mountford had done. I felt like saying, 'Hey guys, it's the other end of me that's injured!'

The doctors decided to keep me in hospital overnight in case I was concussed and I had a big, bossy nurse attending me. I think all the pretty, caring ones had gone home. Anyway, I had to stay awake all night so the nurse kept waking me up and I kept saying, 'Leave me alone.' She'd reply, 'Do as you're told.'

I stopped arguing.

The next day I came out of hospital and I was fine.

A few months later a mate of mine, John Brocas, suggested I give Pre-65 races a go. Pre-65 means the car and engine had to be manufactured before 1965. I'd never really done circuit racing other than kart racing, but I thought it might be a bit of fun, so I suggested we build a car. We found an old Mark 3 Zephyr in Auckland and got to work.

Once I started getting involved I realised that a lot of guys I knew in Tauranga were involved in that class, too. I decided that I wanted to race on the tarseal in the last race at Baypark before they pulled the track to build a residential area. That was a memorable race for me as Baypark had been a big part of my life for years — going there with my dad when I was younger, signwriting some of the race cars, then racing there. Luckily, there are now plans to build a new race track near Tauranga.

John and I worked really hard on the car and had a lot of fun racing it, but the Pre-65 class wasn't as exciting as speedway.

Speedway is extremely fast and full on, you do all your races in one night, whereas in the Pre-65s you race over a weekend. Speedway takes a little bit of getting used to — the intense competition (ideal for me then) and the tightness of the circuit — but it was a motor sport that I enjoyed, and still do enjoy.

As Elaine says, with motor racing, I don't care if I win or lose, it's just being out there and competing that makes me

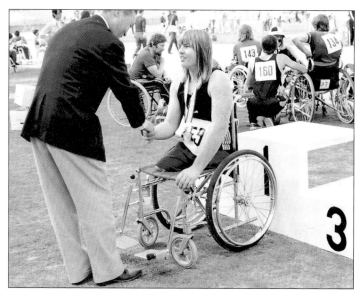

*At just 16 years of age I won silver in the 100 metre sprint
at the FESPIC Games in Oita, Japan, and gold in the
javelin and swimming. It was an amazing experience, and I
still treasure the memory.*

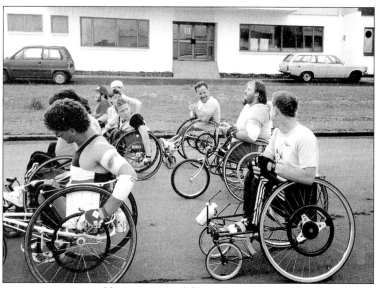

As I got older I progressed from sprints to marathons.

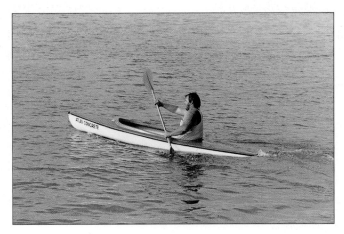

Indoor, outdoor, land or water, I'm happy to try my hand at most sports including kayaking and wheelchair basketball.

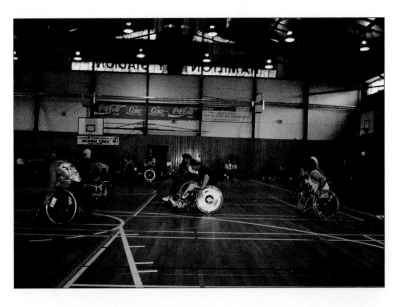

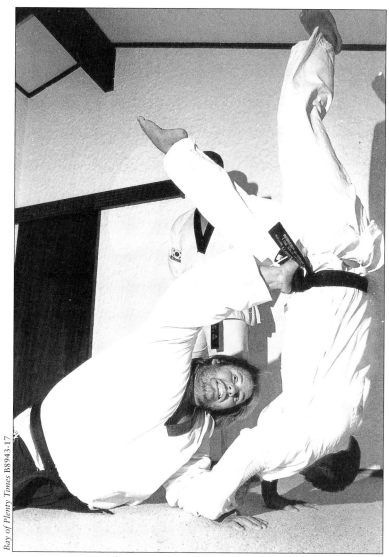

*Mastering the martial art Tae Kwon Do gave me a lot of
confidence. It meant that, should I need to, I could protect
my family and myself.*

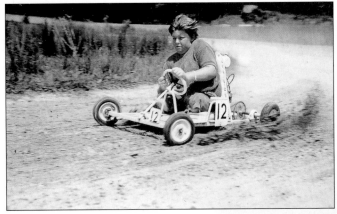

My racing career started
in the go-kart I made
with Dad.

R2D2 aka Tony
Christiansen.

Tearing up the track in
my midget.

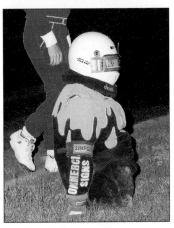

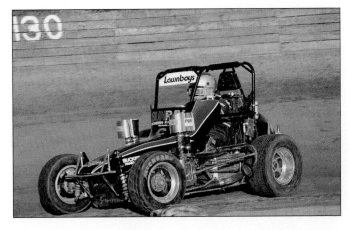

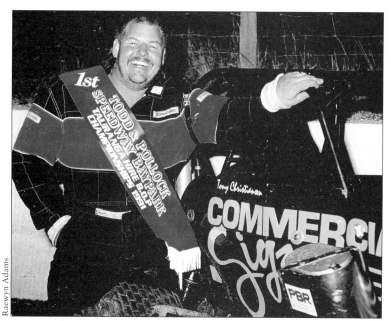

Raewyn Adams

*When you reach one of your goals, it's a great feeling. Here
I am, speedway champion at Baypark, 1991.*

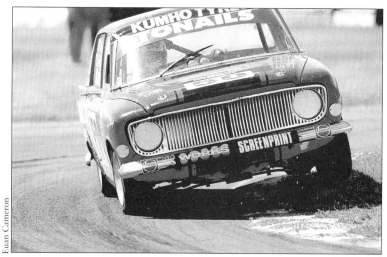

Euan Cameron

My Pre-65 Zephyr, Tonails, taking a corner at speed.

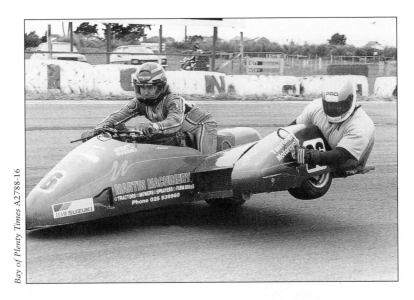

Airborne. Sidecar racing was great fun, but also terrifying.
Flying feels a whole lot safer. My instructor is
Nicola Goodwin.

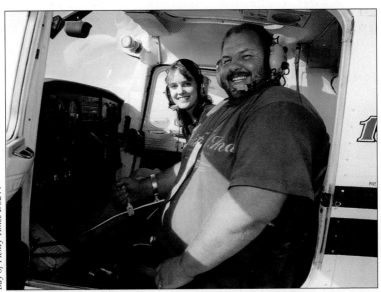

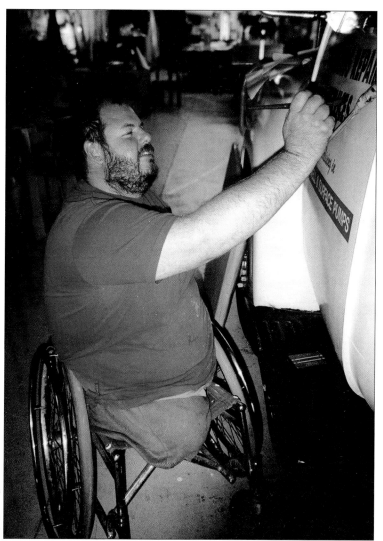

Showing off my signwriting skills.

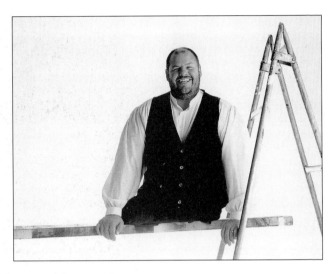

First rule of public speaking: get the audience's attention.
Well, that's one thing I don't have too much difficulty with,
appearing in a wheelchair and climbing up on to my
scaffolding.

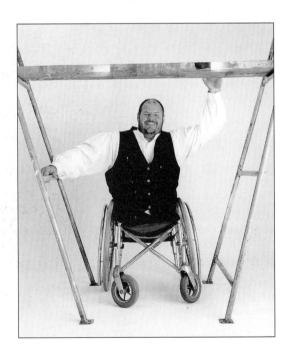

happy. Yeah, I love to win, but even if I come second or third I come off the track yahooing and yelling and screaming. It's the joy of competing that gets my motor running. And that's important with all aspects of life. Why stay in a job if you don't enjoy it: life is too short. Instead, get out there and strive to do what you want to. Sure, it's hard and you can use all sorts of excuses to stop you — kids, a mortgage — but they are *just* excuses stopping you fulfilling your dreams. You're here for a good time, not necessarily a long time. That's why I'm involved in motor racing. It can be a dangerous (and as Elaine reminds me, expensive) sport but it's something I really enjoy, and I'm good at it.

My speedway mates nicknamed me Cannonball, because whenever I had a crash I'd roll away from the car, just like a cannonball. I raced in speedway for two seasons and I had a really good time. I won the six-cylinder class in the championship the first year I competed. My car was just a three-speed automatic, but my aggressive driving got me ahead.

Sometimes, however, my driving caused me a few problems. One night, when I was racing at Western Springs, I had a serious accident. Unfortunately, my parents saw it on television and were very upset as they didn't know how badly injured I was. Elaine was in Tauranga and she was rung by officials and told I was in hospital. She talked to me and I told her I was fine and that a check-up showed I had red eye — a burst blood vessel in my eye — caused when I rolled and my head got shaken around. I was pretty shaken up but looked worse than I was because my eyeball was completely red.

I left speedway racing for a while to concentrate on work, but a mate, Ashley Reid, who crews for me and is an engineer, suggested a couple of years ago that we go back to speedway.

I still had my midget engine, and a guy who wanted it suggested he swap it for a sprint car chassis. So I agreed to that, because I thought the sprint car would be easier to sell than the midget engine, but when I saw the sprint car I thought maybe we should sprint it instead. So we found an engine for it and we raced the sprint car for two seasons, which was awesome. Racing sprint cars can easily be described — the car is seven hundred horsepower and it wants to eat you all the time, it wants to kill you. It was an unbelievable, phenomenal time racing at Western Springs. Ashley was keen to keep racing the sprint car, but the travel back and forth to Auckland during the weekend, and then repairs on the car during the week, got in the way of my public speaking. I didn't have the weekends to myself, as we raced every weekend and weren't back in Tauranga until 3 a.m. on Sunday. I enjoyed the racing but I didn't enjoy the travel.

So we decided to sell the sprint car and move back to the Pre-65 class with a new car. We built the Ford Falcon XP, V8, C4 automatic and last season began racing it. The Pre-65 racing wasn't every weekend and it took a lot less work on the car to keep it up to standard. You'd spend two or three nights a week on the sprint car to get it ready for the next weekend and it was really time that I didn't have. Instead, with the Pre-65, you'd race once every three or four weeks for four months.

From a marketing point of view, a lot of people notice the advertising on my car — Tony Christiansen Presentations — and Pre-65 is a good class, as it's not as stressful as speedway.

Having said that, though, I began speedway racing again near the end of last season, and I realised what a buzz it gave me. But I get a buzz out of any racing and I'd give anything a go once, or twice or even three times. That was the case at a sidecar motorbike meeting at Baypark a few years ago. A friend of mine, Aaron Lovell, had driven sidecars for years, and asked if I wanted to swing for him — ride on the sidecar of the bike and lean out. As I said, I'm willing to give anything a go. I swung for him for a few meetings and it was amazing because you're never so close to dying as when you're millimetres away from the tarseal. One wrong move and you could be dead, and that margin of error was too fine for me. I'd rather be riding the bike than swinging, though my mates reckon they'd have to Velcro my bum to the motorbike seat to keep me on it.

Another motor sport I ventured into was off-road truck racing — a grunty four-wheel-drive, 600 horsepower machine that was capable of speeds up to 130 miles an hour. I raced it with my good friend Euan Cameron, who has an artificial leg. He was driver while I was co-driver/navigator and the joke around the pits was there was only one good leg between us. Euan was supposedly nuts; he had trouble finding people to go with him. The co-driver before me actually vomited half way around the course and said, 'Stop and let me out.'

One race in particular stood out, and I talk about it in my speeches. We were racing at Woodhill Forest, north of Auckland, in the Woodhill 100 race when we hit a rut on Muriwai Beach at 120 miles an hour and end-over-ended three times before the truck landed upside down. I looked across at Euan and asked if he was okay, and he was. Then I looked out the back and saw we had ruptured the fuel tank. Fuel was pouring everywhere, so I told Euan we'd better get out quick. But he had his artificial leg jammed between the accelerator and brake pedals so I undid his prosthesis for him and he hopped away from the truck and we sat by the side of the truck in the sand.

Another competitor saw the accident and rushed back to the pit area and told the officials, 'You'd better get an ambulance down there quick, there's been a horrific accident on the beach front. One guy's got his leg cut off and the other guy's buried up to his waist in sand.'

The officials replied, 'Not those clowns again.'

I have a need to be involved. If it's got an engine in it, point me at it. I want to do rallying next. I want to leave my mark — hey I've tried that, had a go at that, didn't like that. Off-road racing is good, but you get bashed around a bit.

I made my own three-wheeler motorbike when I was a teenager. My mates and I would spend many weekends zooming around on them. Usually one of the guys had a brother who owned a farm, or worked on one, so we'd head out with our bikes and spend hours racing around paddocks. The only problem was the farms were usually quite a way out of Tauranga so we'd have to travel for a while to get to them. It wasn't a simple case of nipping down the road like it was for go-karting.

Off-road biking was a lot of fun. We'd slide around in the mud on the bikes and get completely filthy, but for me that was the half the fun. Then along came the business, children and marriage and they changed those sorts of activities. I didn't have the time or money to spend on 'big boys' toys' and I had to make other activities the priority in my life.

When the kids were a bit older I decided to join my mates in off-roading again, so I bought two old four-wheeler motorbikes and made one good one out of the parts. I sold it and bought a later model with a bigger engine.

Riding was still a lot of fun — getting out and being away from home. On wet days I had a great time being covered in mud — I loved it, I was like a pig in the mud. The group of riders I was with got faster and faster and I'd keep falling off as I didn't have legs to secure me on the bike — I really needed Velcro on my bum.

One incident stood out. A group of mates and I were riding on a local track and I was having a great time speeding around and getting covered in dirt. Then we came around a corner and there was a huge boggy hole in front of us. There were trees down either side so there was no where to go except straight through the mud. Being big and brave, I volunteered to go first.

I hit the bog at great speed, the bike stopped and I kept going — straight over the handlebars. I was sitting in mud up to my waist and my mates were having a huge laugh. I said to them, 'Come on, guys, give me a hand to push the bike out.' As we started to push the bike out, another group of riders came around the corner and stopped. We told them to drive around us and they'd be fine, but instead they took off and went flying into a ditch. I said, 'You wallies, what did you do that for?'

They looked at us and pointed to me and said, 'You're having us on, look how deep it is where he is.'

I climbed out of the mud, and went to the side. The looks on their faces — they couldn't believe it. I jumped on my bike, and took off and when I came back an hour later they were still sitting there staring at the mud.

My need for speed finally got me into serious trouble when I was four-wheel biking a couple of years ago. I was out riding with my mates and they went faster and faster while I tried to keep up. I hit a tree stump as we were going downhill and was flipped over the handlebars. I landed on the ground and the bike kept going and drove over me.

I decided then I was getting too old for that sort of adventure. I went home and told Elaine I wanted to give up four-wheel biking and she asked why, so I showed her my helmet — with a tyre mark across it.

Four-wheel biking had become one of the phases of my life — been there, done that, enough of that, what's next? So I sold the four-wheel bike and bought a jetski.

I had seen guys jetskiing at the beach and I thought it looked fun and it would probably hurt less than falling off my four-wheeler. Also, there were beaches near to my house so it wouldn't be so far to travel as off-roading. So when I found a cheap jetski for sale I bought it and mucked around on it and had a lot of fun. It wasn't big enough for Lucas and I to ride on together as it was a single seater, but I used to drag Lucas behind the jetski in a rubber tube and he loved it — he had a ball.

I decided to sell the single-seater jetski and the four-wheeler and got a bigger jetski, and we went out on it all the time. Lucas and I would go jumping the waves at the beach together. We still have the jetski and, although the kids are older, it's a great family activity — I give the kids a ride on the back and even prop my grandson Houston in front of me and take him for a spin. Jetskiing is one of my pastimes and I find it relaxing, riding the waves and doing tricks.

The great thing about the jetski is that I can put it in the water myself without needing someone to help me, unlike the speedboat. We stopped using the boat when the kids got older, as they weren't so interested hanging around with Mum and Dad and I really needed their help getting it into the lake.

After all the support Tauranga gave me after I accident, I also try to give something back. That includes being a volunteer for the simulated accident training held by the local branch of the St John's Ambulance. Surprisingly, I'm always the 'accident victim' who has lost his legs. Usually the organisers put me in a situation where I have been crushed between objects, like cars. They do a fantastic job of making the accidents look real. They concoct a gooey red substance for blood and create realistic injuries with make-up. One year when I was a volunteer they turned me into a car crash victim who — wild guess — had lost his legs. They poured the 'blood' over my stumps, cut my trousers at the knees and made me lie over the bonnet of a car. The accident looked so real that the two young trainee women nearly fainted when they came across me. Unfortunately, their first aid skills must have been hampered by the sight of my lost limbs, because they put the tourniquet around my waist instead of my stumps. Some years, when I've been a 'victim', the trainees have vomited when they saw me, because the accident looked so realistic.

In 1986 I found a new challenge — martial art. I've always watched kung fu movies and wondered if I could do that. Then I saw a movie where the main character just used two cane walking sticks. I thought, 'If he can do that, then why can't I?'

Nikki was doing Tae Kwon Do lessons at the local hall with her mates. One day I went to pick her up and met her tutor, Allan France. He asked me if wanted I to do some training. I thought, why not? — there's no harm in it and it would be good to challenge myself by trying something new. There were mainly kids in the class and when I started they used to look at me thinking, 'What the heck is he doing here?' I began to learn the blocks and punches and when we were learning round kicks I'd pick myself up and spin around, adapting the move. Tae Kwon Do was great fun. The kids quickly accepted me, and they would spar with me. I became very good at it, and I decided if I wanted to go ahead with this martial art then I'd go for gold — and train towards a black belt.

Nikki gave up soon after I started, probably because her 'old man' was there.

Allan moved to Australia and Kesi O'Neil — another big guy — became the trainer and took me under his wing. He started to give me more one-on-one training because he had several other instructors to look after the kids. He taught me a heck of a lot about Tae Kwon Do and I became quite involved in the sport. After nearly three years of training I went for my grading for my first-degree black belt in Auckland.

This event attracted media attention as it's not often a man with no legs attempts to succeed in a martial art. Mark Sainsbury, a reporter from the TV One current affairs television show, 'Holmes', turned up at the grading session. He was keen to do a story on me getting my black belt, but also wanted to focus on all of my achievements. So Mark and a cameraman spent two days in Tauranga filming my family life and my work and then later added my successful grading in Auckland.

It was a tremendous feeling when I was awarded my first-degree black belt in Tae Kwon Do. Once again, I was really breaking out of the mould of what a 'disabled' person should do.

'You can't do that,' people would when I told them I was learning Tae Kwon Do, 'you don't have any legs.' Surprise! I can do. See, it's all about people's perceptions. What do these people want me to do? Sit at home in my wheelchair and moan about not having any legs? Not this fella, thank you very much.

Once I had my black belt I began to teach and that was great fun because of the kids' perception: 'Hey, you've got no legs, you can't do that.' I proved to be an inspiration to them, showing them that they shouldn't listen to people who try to tell them that things can't be done.

In 1989 I represented New Zealand in a demonstration Tae Kwon Do team that went to Western Samoa. It went very well; people there had never seen a person with no legs compete, and they were impressed, especially as I was throwing Kesi, who weighed 150 kilograms, over my shoulder.

The next year I decided to go for my second-degree black belt. I kept training, kept going to the classes and again my goal became an important part of my life. I achieved my aim, but I decided it was time to move on and do other things. I still do a little bit of Tae Kwon Do — just mucking around — as it's something that you can always go back to. Tae Kwon Do gave me a lot of confidence. I've always felt vulnerable without legs as I felt I would be at a disadvantage in a fight.

But Tae Kwon Do taught me that I actually had an advantage over other people. If someone is going to kick you, they are standing on only one leg. As soon as they are on one leg they're off balance, and as soon as they are off balance they are yours. So I can take people down pretty easily, and I know what to look for. From the confidence point, I know I could protect my family and myself if I needed to. In practice, I have used a walking cane as a weapon, and that hook can be pretty dangerous. You can hook someone around the neck, pull them around the leg and tip them off balance, trip them, or hook them between the buttocks or around the groin. It's a very good weapon, and it's legal to carry. Sure, it's not going to be a lot of good against a gun. But I believe that if I *was* in a confrontational situation, I'd sooner walk away (or in my case, wheel away) than do something — Tae Kwon Do has taught me discipline.

In the early '90s I entered an able-bodied weightlifting competition in Tauranga and with my big build I competed in the bench press. I won it with a lift of 220 kilograms, but I was disqualified. I asked why, and the organisers said one of the other competitors brought to their attention the rule that all competitors must wear the correct footwear.

Darn, I must have forgotten to put my shoes on that day.

Sure, I could have ranted and raved about how unfair that was, but I don't like confrontations so I let it go. Besides, I felt that the complaining competitor wanted to win more than I did — no matter how unfairly.

I'm always after a new challenge — once I've set a goal and achieved it I've got to move on and that's how I created aviation history in New Zealand.

For many years I've mucked around with radio-controlled planes as I've always had a fascination with flight. When I was

13, I flew to the Ardmore air show in a friend's dad's airplane and that's where my love of flying started. My mate's dad let me fly his plane for a bit and I knew then that I was hooked and one day I'd fly by myself. But, in the meantime, I stuck with model airplanes. I started to build rubber band-propelled planes and I'd climb up a ladder and throw them off my parents' roof. See, not having legs didn't stop me doing typical boys' stuff. A mate and I used to make the flying more challenging by shooting the airplanes with a slug gun.

Mum was not amused.

Later on, I got involved in radio-controlled planes. I stole one of Danie's Barbie dolls, put it in one of the planes, and every time it crashed I'd blame it on the woman driver!

A few of my friends were involved in radio-controlled planes and I enjoyed building and flying my own planes and doing aerobatics with them. Phil Hooker, a pilot with Air New Zealand who lived in Tauranga, was also interested in radio-controlled planes. But he had a few crashes in the planes (model ones, not Air New Zealand's, thank goodness) and he didn't have the knowledge to repair them so I offered to fix them for him. To pay me back for the work I did on his radio-controlled planes, Phil suggested he take me, Danie and Lucas for a flight around Tauranga at night in his small plane. The kids really loved the flight but they didn't realise that I was flying the airplane the whole time! I think once you know how to fly one thing you become a natural at knowing aircraft. Phil was using the rudder and I was using the hand control. I landed the plane — it was a beautiful, calm night so it was easy.

Shortly after that Phil approached me to paint some signs for him, as he was starting his own flight school at Tauranga airport. Then, mucking around on the Internet one night, he got some information on wheelchair-bound flyers in America, disabled people flying with hand controls. Phil asked me if I wanted to learn to fly — the publicity would be good for him. He would sponsor me as far as the solo stage, and then I'd have to pay for the rest to go for my private pilot's licence.

It took me thirteen hours to fly solo, and a total of fifty hours to get my licence. But on 24 March 1998, I created New Zealand aviation history by being the first person to learn and fly solo with a disability. There are several other disabled pilots in New Zealand, but they were pilots before they were injured.

It was an amazing day for me.

On a training flight with Phil, I lined up on the runway, took off, did a complete circuit and a perfect landing. Phil told me to pull over to the side of the runway and said to me, 'Tony, you're ready to fly solo.' He got out of the plane and walked away and he never looked back. I taxied the plane around, lined up on the runway, pushed the throttle forward, and climbed to 1000 feet. On the downward leg I did my radio calls and pre-landing checks, and I put 10 degrees of flap on the wings. That made the plane wallow a bit and I quickly looked towards the instructor's seat — but Phil wasn't there any more. There was no one there to take over if things went wrong. I descended the aircraft to 600 feet, put 30 degrees of flap on, and the plane shuddered again. Still Phil wasn't there, still no one to take over. I landed the plane — one of my best landings — and in doing so, I flew into the aviation history books.

By gaining my licence I achieved another goal, and that taught me that you should take every opportunity that is offered. Phil and I were in a win-win situation, but it still took courage, commitment and patience to get out there and learn to fly.

People have suggested I train for my instrument licence so I can fly by myself and even fly to my seminars. One of the problems is that if the weather is dodgy and I have to fly out that day to give a speech, then I could be stuck in Tauranga. An instrument licence would help in some situations, but on a commercial flight I have an even better chance of getting to my destination.

I'm still keen on flying and I try to keep my hours up by flying once or twice a month, but it is an expensive hobby.

My attitude is to make use of every opportunity and that has shown through throughout my adult life. I've tried lots of sports — from squash to tennis to basketball. I still play wheel-chair basketball, but it was playing squash that amazed most people. I played in the early 1980s with mates every Wednesday to keep fit — and I was a lot fitter then than I am now. I used to shuffle around on my bum to hit the ball; I could move very quickly, and that surprised people.

I carried on with some of my sports because the opportunities were there. With squash, what opportunities are there for a guy with no legs? They don't play squash in the Disabled Games and they don't have a disabled competition in squash. It was great fun, something to do, but that was as far as it would go. It was the same with Tae Kwon Do. I could have got one more grading and become an instructor or a referee, but where to from there?

I also competed in three marathons. As I was so strong in the arms, I was able to wheel along at great pace and finish in good times. In 1980 I competed in the Fletcher marathon raced around Lake Rotorua. Wheelchair competitors had been in-cluded a couple of times but had been stopped for a few years because of the difficulties involved, like passing runners. The first year they let us start five minutes after the runners, which wasn't a problem. But with the improvements in wheelchair technology, especially the invention of the three-wheel chair, we became faster, and tried to overtake runners. They then let us start five minutes before the runners, which seemed to solve the problem.

In 1980 I finished in three hours, 58 minutes and in 1981 in three hours, 20 minutes; able-bodied runners were doing it in three hours. It was a hard event, as the terrain wasn't flat and the hills took it out of me. An easier marathon was the local Tauranga race in 1984, where I also finished in a good time, but by then I was beginning to focus on work and motor sport.

I also took my love of flying quite literally and did a tandem parachute dive. It was an exhilarating experience — being thrown from a plane and free-falling away, then the parachute kicking in and floating to the earth. I loved it.

People's perception is very strange — 'Hey, you've got no legs, you can't play squash', or, 'He's got a sense of humour and jokes about having no legs.' It's just perception. I like to play on that when people ask me how I lost my legs — the story changes regularly.

When Elaine, the kids and I were holidaying in Hawaii a few years ago, we were sitting on the beach and some kids came up and asked how I lost my legs. I pointed to the sea and said, 'I was out there swimming and the sharks took them.'

When we went on a glass-bottom boat in Hawaii a guy came up to me and said, 'Did you lose your legs in 'Nam, mate?' I said yes, but later I complained to Elaine that I was too young to be in Vietnam. I was in a rough pub a while ago with a mate when some bikies came in and they got talking to me and asked how I lost my legs. I said, 'I came off my motorbike, man.' Boy, was my street cred high then. See, it's all perception.

Phil Hooker, who taught me how to fly, is New Zealand's most highly qualified flying instructor. An Air New Zealand pilot for twelve years, he is also a B category glider pilot, operations officer for all microlights in New Zealand, and flies power parachutes, amphibian planes, helicopters and gyrocopters. Phil owns the country's fastest growing flight centre, training airline and recreational pilots.

I first saw Tony doing a tandem sky dive at Tauranga airport, then I met him through the model aircraft club. I kept crashing my model planes and I'd go round to his place and he'd have to rebuild them. He taught me how to fly model airplanes then we got to talking about flying.

Tony remembered reading a story when he was a teenager about a paraplegic man in the States who learned how to fly. I told him I had a flying school so why didn't he come and have a look at it. On the Internet, I found out about an organisation called International Wheelchair Aviators. I emailed them and got some information about flying for the disabled. Then I found out about hand controls that are connected to the rudder pedal, and even phoned a guy in the States about it. At the time I couldn't afford to buy the $2,000 kit from America, but a year after Tony and I first talked about it I was able to purchase the kit and we started training.

I had also read in a magazine about a paraplegic New Zealander who had a disabled kit. I rang the Civil Aviation Authority to track him down and eventually found him in Christchurch. As I flew for Air New Zealand, the next time I was in Christchurch I met him and he showed me the kit. Although he was a pilot before his accident he'd had to go through the CAA red tape to fly again, so he had paved the way for Tony.

Training Tony was no different to training any other student once the hand control kit went on. It was a bonus that

Tony had been involved in aviation for a while — he'd been up in a glider, a helicopter, and had a friend, Frank Wright, at Tauranga airport who resorted aircraft. So Tony knew a lot about aviation; also, he flew model aircraft and that's a lot harder than the real thing.

Mine was the only place in the country that catered for disabled pilots and Tony was a breeze to teach — a natural. He went solo a little bit earlier than other guys mainly because he flew model aircraft and he understood the technical side of flying.

His medical was an interesting one — I told my doctor that I was bringing a guy with no legs for a medical. When Tony and I entered the doctor's surgery the receptionist was sitting behind a high desk and could only see me.

I said to her, 'Hi, Tony Christiansen for a medical.'

She replied, 'Take a seat, Mr Christiansen.'

I said, 'No, it's for Tony.'

The receptionist said, 'Where is he? Is he coming in?'

And I said, 'No, he's right here' pointing to Tony below me.

She leaned over the counter and nearly had a heart attack.

Tony did the normal medical, though he had a few problems with some parts of the test — like standing on one leg — and the weight to height ratio didn't match up. For Tony's weight he had to be seven feet tall.

I didn't treat him any differently than my other students and he certainly brought some colour to the place, especially compared to the young guys. They'd be complaining about not having any money and generally moaning and Tony, even back then, was pretty motivated. He'd say to them, 'Look at me. What the heck's wrong with you? Get off your bum.'

We had a prize-giving evening for people going solo and one of the students, who was quite big and only 21, had been drinking and gave Tony a hard time about his black belt in Tae Kwon Do.

He said to Tony, 'What the heck can you do? A black belt and you can't even kick anyone. I could come and overpower you and you couldn't do a damn thing.'

Tony said, 'Yes I could.'

The guy said, 'You're just short and fat, what can you do?'

And within a blink of an eye Tony rolled over, hit the guy's legs and knocked him flat on the floor. Tony then sat on him, put his arms on his hips and replied, 'What were you saying?'

When Tony went solo it was big news in the civil aviation industry. I was very proud of him. I'm proud of all of my students, but with Tony I was especially proud because he was a mate and it was a special day.

When Tony flies now he puts the kit in himself. Originally we tried to put the hand controls in for Tony, but he said he should do it. So he installs them and we do some of the pre-take-off checks, like getting up on the wings, then he takes off and we forget about him. When he comes back, we make sure his wheelchair is near to where his aircraft will land — but only if we're heading out there. He doesn't want any special favours.

He could have his pilot's licence now, as he's passed all of the tests bar one; unfortunately, his speaking engagements prevent him from sitting the test. With a bit of revision he could get his pilot's licence easily. Once Tony gets his pilot's licence he can go for a commercial pilots' licence, then train up to be an instructor. I've told him I'd be quite happy to employ him as an instructor in my school.

He's talked about circumnavigating New Zealand or a trans-Tasman flight, and when he gets the time I'm sure he'll do it.

CHAPTER SEVEN
MINDING MY OWN BUSINESS

*'My goal was to own my own business by the time I
was 30 — I achieved that three years early.'*

BY 1985 I had left Commercial Signs and was working for
another signwriting company in Tauranga. I was quite happy
at the new company but I still had a goal — owning my own
signwriting business.

Kathy Styles, co-owner of Commercial Signs, my old company, rang up one day and said her then husband Lance wanted
out of the business. When she asked if I was interested in buying his half share of Commercial Signs, I leapt at the chance. It
was a great opportunity for me. I was 27 years old. My goal
was to own my own business by the time I was 30 — I achieved
that three years early.

But it was a dramatic change for me, going back there. I
was a former work-mate on Friday, the boss on Monday. I've
always tried to be a friendly person and I like interacting with
people and enjoy other people's company. I used to have Friday night drinks with the other guys at Commercial Signs and
went out with them socially. But on the Monday morning when
I started work the whole attitude towards me changed. Instead of 'Hey, Tony', it was 'Yes, boss'.

I took it to heart and wanted to be friends with them. But it wasn't long before the harsh reality set in — I couldn't be their employer and friends with them as well. It was my business, my money, I'd put a lot in to it — the mortgage, my house — and I had a lot of responsibility. I found sometimes that's where conflict arose — because my workers were quite happy to settle for second best or took a 'She'll be right' attitude, and I believed that wasn't what I was there for and neither was it what I wanted to give my customers. Hey, I had been one of those staff who said, 'She'll be right', and 'What's the boss whingeing about'. But it's not until you become the employer that you realise the difference and I was pretty quick to pick up on it — you couldn't be on the same level as those guys.

I'd still have beers with the guys on Friday night after work but this time I was buying the beer instead of drinking it, so I'd watch how much we'd drink! I always believed that the Friday night social gathering was great and I said to my employees that when we're having a beer they could say anything to me — and they did. I also had a policy at work that my door was always open — if they needed to talk to me about anything then they could because it was important to discuss any potential conflicts.

I always felt I had some business skills — I was good with dealing with customers and I could see where and how I wanted my company to grow. But I didn't think I knew it all, so I attended a few personal development conferences — Success Motivation International (SMI) courses and the Dale Carnegie seminars — and they helped me with my business. I had this massive responsibility, and I had to make it work and make a success out of it. Not being successful was never going to be an option for me, so I tried to do everything I could to succeed.

I started with a one-day seminar in Auckland. One of my customers, Lawrence O'Toole, had a company called Creative

Training, and as payment for doing some signs for him, he gave Kathy and me tickets to see Joseph Basich, a business guru from Australia. I learnt a lot in that one day; that's where I got enthusiastic about public speaking, because I saw the magic that he had and his ability to capture people's attention — he certainly captured mine.

He walked in and said, 'Good morning' and then, 'Goodbye' and walked out. There were two hundred people sitting in the room, a few of them from Tauranga, and we were looking at each other, bewildered. Everyone was getting restless after five minutes when he hadn't reappeared. Then he walked back in and said, 'Thank you for coming. You are here, you paid to be here, and for that I thank you, but if you don't listen that's all you're going to get, "Good morning" and "Goodbye".'

All of a sudden he had everyone's attention.

I listened and listened and I thought some of the stuff was rubbish — he was from that older school that said to be successful you had to wear a tie, a blue suit and shirt and have no facial hair. Well, I had a beard so I failed straight away and I didn't have legs either — I was in real trouble. But I got so much out of the seminar: I learnt about communicating and about service; he said that without your clients, you're nothing, so you must pay attention to what your client wants; and I discovered I had to decide what I was, a manager or a worker. I'd tried to be a worker-manager and it didn't work. I was very hands on, paintbrush in hand. I had twenty years' experience and I loved signwriting. I went from being foreman at Commercial Signs and working seven hours a day signwriting and one hour managing, to seven hours managing and one hour signwriting. Then I found that the signwriting wasn't even an option, because though I could use my creativity I had to use my workers as my hands. The people I had working for me suddenly had to be my tools, and I became the supplier of the work, because if I didn't go out and do my job — marketing — then there was no work for my staff.

Then Kathy bought an SMI personal development course — audio tapes and a workbook schedule — but she wasn't interested in it so I gave it a go and really enjoyed it. It consisted of simple day-to-day planning and affirmations. I've still got the tapes and I still play them in my car. The tapes were learning tools — like verbal workbooks — and I enjoyed listening to them. The tapes didn't motivate me, because I'm a very motivated person to begin with, but they helped me focus and let me look at something in a different way. The course also taught me about communicating with my staff — simple things about dealing with disputes. Most bosses deal with their staff with a heavy-handed, overbearing attitude — negative, negative, negative. Instead, you should say, 'You're so good at this, you're really good at this, you could do a bit of work on that area, and we can work on that, but you have a few problems with this side of things.'

We are in a world where we berate people into submission so they will do what we want them to do because of the fear of losing their job. The first thing bosses say is usually, 'Do you like your job, or don't you like working here?' Instead of saying, 'I enjoy having you here, it's great and I think we get on really well, but I think there are issues we need to look at.' I know what I would like to hear. The other way is just using fear tactics.

W. Mitchell, an American motivational speaker who was badly burned then paralysed in two separate accidents, said, 'It's not what happens to you, it's what you do about it.' In one way I don't agree with that, because when you say, 'It's not what happens to you' it means you spend your life reacting to things instead of making them happen. Why do we have to always be reacting to situations? Why is it that only adversity will motivate you — or inhibit you? Who said you can only challenge yourself if you face a crisis in your life? Or make life-changing decisions when you hit a climax in your life? Why is it that we allow mediocrity to let our goals slip by? The mentality is that you should stick to what you know best and don't push the boundaries.

I believe that you should make things happen in your life — just do it.

I like to believe that's what I did in my business life — I went out and made it happen.

I loved my job and that reflected in my work — I was great at dealing with people, not just workers but clients, and I was good at my job. Through my personality and drive Commercial Signs increased business both locally and in the Bay of Plenty and Waikato regions. By the late 1980s and early 1990s Commercial Signs was the biggest signwriting business in the Bay of Plenty because I was going out there and getting the work.

Kathy and I went through the business roller-coaster of getting more work and more people; in the end, we doubled our workshop staff to twelve. But more staff does not always mean more profit, and we found out our outgoings were too much. Our optimum level was seven staff — we made more money with seven than with twelve because of the overheads, but it took us a year to find that out. This was before the age of computers, when information on incoming and outgoing finances became more readily available. You have to have a regular accounts payable tally to know what your situation is. But before computers we'd have a balance for a month and then we'd split that in to days to gain a reasonable indication of where we were. By the time I finished with the company I could get a weekly, sometimes daily, report from the computer.

One of the things I enjoyed about my job was being out there, climbing ladders and painting signs. I became well-known in Tauranga as 'the signwriter with no legs'. I even had mail addressed to me like that — and it found its way to me.

There were some funny incidents while I was signwriting up scaffolding. People would walk past and there would be three of us up the scaffolding and only two pairs of legs. The person would stop, look again and then be totally confused. The most memorable occasion was when we were painting the sign for a shoe shop and there I was, a signwriter with no legs, painting the sign 'Hannahs Footwear'. Someone took a photo and sent it to the signwriters' magazine. Another time I was doing a sign for a bank's front window and I was having a break, lying down on the scaffolding and leaning my head on my elbow. A woman came into the bank, went up to the manager and told him she didn't like the big gnome in the window.

But in the early 1990s there were major changes in the signwriting industry. Out went hand-painted signs and in came vinyl-cutting technology. Commercial Signs was one of the first signwriting businesses in the North Island to get a vinyl-cutting computer. It had an illustrator programme with different letter styles. Big rolls of self-adhesive vinyl would run through the special cutter. This cut the vinyl with a very sharp knife and you'd just peel the back off and you'd have the lettering. It had the advantage of being a very quick process and it saved a person having to hand paint a job then wait for the paint to dry.

One of the perceptions people had about vinyl cutting was that because it was computer generated, and it was quick, it must be saving a lot of money in labour costs. But the start-up cost was $35,000 for the computer hardware, software, plotters and cutters. Then you had to have $10,000 worth of different coloured vinyl in stock. In the old days, I had about $100 worth of paint pots on the shelves of the workshop, my brushes, and my experience. All of a sudden, to be competitive in the market, we had to have the $35,000 computer, we had to have the vinyls in stock, then we had to have an operator because I didn't have the skills to run the machinery. I had to employ people to become vinyl cutters and applicators rather than skilled signwriters, which changed the industry a lot.

Then our marketing changed. We had to go out and look for markets for the vinyl printing, like real estate companies with all their sale signs, auction signs and hoardings. That realty work became a huge market for Commercial Signs. We became known as the 'get it in, get it done, get it out' company, because of our fast turn-around time. Tauranga was opening up in the early 1990s, with lots of subdivisions being created, and nearby Papamoa was being developed as well. At one time there were sixty-four subdivisions in the local area, and we did the signage for forty-seven of them. We also covered anything repetitious, like truck and trailer fleet signage. Then illuminated signs became a major part of the company.

Our next major purchase was a machine that could cut lettering out of wood, steel, aluminium and polystyrene. We used to cut all this out with a jigsaw, but now you could just put it down and the computer would cut it out for you. Although this was a $100,000 machine as opposed to a $300 jigsaw, you had to have it because that's what people demanded.

With this computer technology, a lot of large corporations moved all their operations to their main offices. So instead of having a guy in Tauranga doing the signage for the local branch of a large brewery company, the brewery would get all their signs nationwide done in Auckland by a large signwriting company. Commercial Signs had to adjust to that too — we had to go out and find that business. Soon the company became the main suppliers of signage for big businesses in the middle North Island because we had the gear for it. To boost that, we began installing signs produced by large companies in Auckland. Suddenly I needed fewer and fewer signwriters, or people with the same hands-on skills that I had. Instead we needed builders, and people with aluminium experience, and applicators — people who could stick on vinyl over moulded shapes and such things. That was a shame, because I felt that we lost a lot of skill. The up side was that these times showed how successful Commercial Signs had become around Tauranga. It was great for me to drive around and see our signs all over town — I was very proud. It also created more work for us because people want to deal with successful companies. I believe that this was one of the reasons that we did well — success breeds success. If you hang around with successful people, then some of the success is likely to rub off on you. So, with that in mind, I always made sure I had the biggest signwriters ad in the Yellow Pages; people would think that Commercial Signs must be very successful to warrant such a big ad. Although the cost was $3,000 per ad, one job would pay for it.

In mid-1995 things were changing again at Commercial Signs, this time between Kathy and me. Kathy had bought a 10-acre kiwi fruit orchard with her new partner Stu, and her direction and focus in life had changed. I could see she lacked enthusiasm for her work. But I wanted to carry on being successful, and I didn't know how the company was going to work without Kathy being a part of it. There was only one way to find out. So I asked her questions. How long did she intend to stay? What were her intentions with the orchard and Commercial Signs? She didn't really know.

The orchard was going really well for her and Stu but they needed two people working full time to make it successful, while I needed her full time at Commercial Signs. And while her focus in life had changed, so too had mine — I wanted to become the sole owner, to do things myself and make my own business decisions.

At this stage, Kathy wasn't willing to make a decision; and then, when we got down to numbers, there was some conflict over how much Kathy wanted to sell her share of the company for. I felt that, although we were shareholders in the company, I earned more on the production side. Whether that was right or wrong, I don't know. She did the administration and all the office work and when I did take over, and before Elaine helped out, I did have to do a lot of work that I never really knew was needed, like bill paying. I looked at a balance sheet at the end of the day and it always looked good to me, so I never asked Kathy any questions. But I felt the balance sheet reflected the work we did out in the workshop, rather than what was done in administration. I am not criticising Kathy's work, but I knew I could employ someone to replace her.

Kathy sold me the business in December 1995, six months after the initial suggestion. In the beginning, Elaine wasn't very enthusiastic about my taking over the business from Kathy because we had to borrow more money. But I believed we were always going to be in debt, it was just the level of debt that varied. To make money you have to spend money. Elaine's attitude was the opposite; she worried about paying back a big mortgage. But buying the business was something I knew we could do successfully and Elaine was reassured that the business would pay the extra mortgage.

With Kathy leaving, it meant I had to do so much more myself. I worked from seven in the morning to seven at night instead of my previous hours of eight to four thirty. I would be so busy answering questions during the day and having to be available to people — not only staff but clients and suppliers — that I had a lot more administrative work after hours. I used to do invoices during the day when Kathy was working, but when she left I couldn't do that any more, I had to do it at night. But I had a policy of not doing that at home; I did it a couple of times, and it didn't work for a number of reasons. Work was work and home was home. And there were distractions at home, too, only different — the kids, the phone. And I had all the information I needed in files at work — how much paint was used, how much tape and so on. I found it easier at the end of the work day to lock my office door and spend an hour and a half doing administrative work.

Another major change after Kathy left was the responsibility I faced. The whole structure had to change — I had to become the point at which the buck stopped. It was like that before, but it was an even bigger buck when I bought out Kathy.

I always seemed to be borrowing more money to do things — buy computers, buy out Kathy — and just when I was getting ahead there'd be that need to borrow more money to do something else. But these were always steps in the direction I wanted to go — steps towards owning my own business, being the sole responsible owner, making it go in the direction I wanted.

I looked for different opportunities when Kathy left, instead of pursuing small but frequent jobs like the signs for real estate companies. I knew we had the capability to handle big contracts, so why should that work go out of town to Auckland companies? So we changed, and we got that work by knocking on doors and using opportunities, like the tender for the Mainzeal contract. The tender was advertised for signage for a $2.5 million carpark that was being built in Tauranga. We were contacted by Mainzeal to quote for it along with two Auckland signwriting companies. There were lots of phone calls and faxes between myself and John Palmer from Mainzeal's Hamilton office. We sent the tender through and we got the job, so he came to Tauranga to meet me for the first time.

I bet from our conversations that he had an image of me as a six foot two rugby player.

I knew he was coming in at lunchtime and I was sitting in my office where I could see the front door when he arrived. He had on a blue T-shirt with Mainzeal on it, so I wheeled out of the office, went up to him and stuck my hand out. I was between him and my receptionist and he looked straight over my head to my receptionist and said, 'I'm John Palmer from Mainzeal, I'm here to see Tony.'

I looked up at him and said, 'Hi John, I'm Tony.'

He looked down at me and there was this shocked look on his face. I could see by his eyes he was thinking, 'Bugger, what have I done? How is this guy going to do my $2.5-million carpark? He's got no legs. Should we tell him?' I could see in an instant that I only had thirty seconds to restore that confidence. Business schools say you have ninety seconds to make an impression on a person when you first meet them — I have thirty. And you only have one chance at that first impression. So I had to prove to John that choosing the company and me was the best option for Mainzeal. I did that by confidence.

I said, 'Hi John, pleased to meet you. Thanks for the opportunity, would you like to come and see our workshop? Come through and see our facilities.' He came, and when he saw the guys and all the equipment all of a sudden this weight lifted off his shoulders.

It was the same with most of the clients when I met them for the first time. I'd jump out the back of the van and wheel up to them wearing my T-shirt with 'Commercial Signs' on it. And the look on their faces was, 'He's got no legs, how am I going to tell him that I've got a 15-metre wall to signwrite?' So I'd jump out of my chair onto the ground, or climb up something saying, 'So, you're looking for the sign to go about here?'

Or I'd bring a ladder out of the van. Or I'd have the boys with me and we'd get a ladder off the truck and climb up it. Those sort of tactics. And all of a sudden the clients were reassured.

It's all about how clients perceive me. I have to quickly prove to them that it doesn't matter that I don't have legs, I'm capable of doing the job — not only the physical side, like climbing ladders, but also the technical side of creating their sign. People's perception is always a tough one, as even in today's society a lot of people think that if you have a physical challenge then you're mentally retarded too. Strangers come up to me and speak slowly — like I'm mentally challenged. Or else they speak loudly to me. I feel like saying to them, 'I'm in a wheelchair, not deaf.' So people's perception is something I enjoy trying to change because they look at me and think, 'You can't climb ladders, you don't have any legs.'

I think, 'Who decided that? Where did that come into the script?'

And we used perception in the business in other ways. When Commercial Signs was originally split up, the signwriting side of the business was sold to Lance and Kathy and the screenprinting to Ray; the two businesses still worked out of the same building. This was good when I owned the business, as people's perception was that it was one large company and people could come to Commercial Signs and get everything done. We never told them that it was two separate businesses, even when I moved the business two doors down. If people needed screenprinting done I'd say to them to go to our other office. Again, it's perception — all people saw was a whole block in central Tauranga that said 'Commercial Signs'.

I rarely had disputes with clients over cost because Commercial Signs gave them good service at a responsible cost and most of the time we let them know what it was going to cost before we started the work. That is something I learnt quickly

— never let clients leave without letting them know what their job is going to cost. The women in the front office were taught enough about the work so that they could give an estimate for a sign over the phone. Say someone wanted an eight-by-four sign and I wasn't there to take the phone call, the receptionist could tell them that it would cost approximately $350. The worst thing you can say is 'I don't know'. Never, ever admit that you don't know. Because if you don't know — who does? The client doesn't give a hoot if you don't know, all they want is an answer.

When I bought the business, we had two women working in the office, one part-time, but when the full-timer left Elaine began working in the office a couple of mornings a week because her back injury prevented her working as a chef. She started doing reception work and taking orders, doing a few small signs, and getting to know more about the business. Soon she was in charge of chasing up payment of bills — and she was good at it. Very good, as she doesn't mind confrontations. Our bank manager was very impressed with how the business was going and with Elaine's contribution. Later on, when we decided to sell the business, the bank manager told us that he didn't know if Commercial Signs would do quite so well without us, as Tony Christiansen was Commercial Signs. Clients knew me, and knew they'd get a good job from me. That was a great honour. It showed that I had succeeded in my aim to run a top-rate business.

I also passed on my signwriting skills to my apprentices. But usually, when they came out of their apprenticeship, they stayed with me six months and then left to go overseas. I always encouraged them to travel, but it was tough. When you teach someone a trade the expectation is that they will stay with you for a few years afterwards to pay back the investment you put into them. I always like to pass on my skills, though.

But things were changing at Commercial Signs, and I began to realise the challenge wasn't there any more and I needed a new focus. Two guys who worked for me left, bought their own vinyl-cutting computer, and took some of my clients. Then, suddenly, lots of people were buying the computers — architects, guys who put racing stripes on cars and so on. The computer technology really changed the signwriting business and it affected Commercial Signs' turnover. If I had to compete with these smaller guys, I'd have to down-size and change the way I worked, following the smaller guys into their market.

This re-emphasises another point I've made — if you don't believe in it, don't do it. And I didn't believe in signwriting any more, which was sad, as I always imagined I'd retire as a signwriter and pass the business over to my son. But it shows you that your focus can change.

However, I had found my new passion and challenge — to be the best inspirational speaker in New Zealand, and eventually one of the best in the world.

Signwriting had taken me on a business roller coaster and I'd got to the point where I thought, 'Where is this going to take me? Am I still going to be here in ten years' time? I've got this other opportunity here.' And I saw inspirational speaking as another opportunity in life. Where it is going to take me, I don't know, but I've never been one to be scared of taking an opportunity. Life is simply a whole series of opportunities — where you go depends on which ones you want to take, what rewards you are after, and what size risk you are prepared to take. That's what life is all about.

Frustration had begun to build up at Commercial Signs. We had twelve to fourteen staff and all the difficulty that goes with that — clients not paying on time and staff hassles. One day in particular changed my life. We had just paid a whole lot of GST, we were up to date, and I was sitting in my office thinking everything was fine. Then Elaine came up with a letter from Inland Revenue saying we owed a further $3,000 for something else. From what I understood, it was IRD's cock-up and they were trying to get me to pay a penalty on it. I got so angry and so wild that I said to Elaine, 'Forget it, I'm not doing this any more.'

Elaine agreed with me, so I rang a real estate agent — one who specialised in businesses — that afternoon and asked him to come and see us. He said, 'I'd love to list your business.' He asked me how much I wanted for it. I wrote the amount on a piece of paper and slipped it to him — I wanted a good deal of money for the business, hundreds of thousands of dollars. He mulled over it, so I showed him how much I was making and my GST receipts for the past six months and he perked up a bit. He had a quick look around and then came back to my office. He said, 'There are people out there who are in the market for a business like yours, but I reckon it will take three to six months to sell.'

I signed up with him and within three days he had sold the business.

He brought one interested party through twenty-four hours after I signed up, then the next day came with two more. Then he appeared with a contract. I looked at him and laughed and told him, 'I told you how much I wanted and this isn't it.' I dropped the price slightly, put a highlighter pen through the new price, sent it back to him and said, 'Don't come back to me unless you have that amount signed.' He came back that afternoon with it signed.

There I was, my business sold within three days instead of six months, and I was thinking, 'What am I doing?'

Elaine continued to worry about whether we were doing the right thing, however. Who would sell a business like ours to go into speaking, an occupation that *might* give you a lot of work but might not? To appease her, not only did I hassle my speaking agents for more bookings, but I also agreed with the new owner that I'd stay on as works manager and receive a wage but not have the hassle of running the place.

With the money from the sale of the business, we cleared the mortgage and all the bills and were sitting pretty. But I didn't like the way things were being run at Commercial Signs and, besides, I was getting busier on the speaking circuit. I had told the new owners when I took on the job that my priority was my public speaking, and they didn't like it that I wasn't available for certain signwriting jobs. I talked to one of the guys I worked with about what I should do — chuck in the job and focus on speaking or stay as I was? He gave me some great advice — only I would know if it was the right time to focus on speaking.

And I knew that it was.

I left Commercial Signs for good and began my path towards being the best inspirational speaker in the world.

CHAPTER EIGHT

'UNACCUSTOMED AS I AM TO PUBLIC SPEAKING . . .'

'If you set goals and try your hardest to succeed, then you will . . . You should take every opportunity that comes your way.'

MY NEW career path began through my friend Lawrence O'Toole, from Creative Training. He asked me if I'd speak to a group of long-term unemployed doing a course he was running in Tauranga. He wanted me to talk not only from the point of view of being an employer, but also from the 'challenge' side. I found the group hard work as they were so unmotivated, but after speaking to them for over an hour I got some great responses and later on some of them wrote me letters. I spoke to them once a week and developed my skills in speaking to groups of people — especially people who didn't want to be there to listen.

Lawrence was in Rotary so I spoke to them — for a free meal — and my confidence grew from talking to one person, to ten people, to a hundred people. In the end, size didn't daunt me.

I did a Success Motivation International course in personal leadership, then followed that up with a course in business management, and because of my success I became an SMI Gold

Member. That was determined by my business progress during the year and it was also recognition from SMI. Being a Gold Member meant speaking at an awards evening at the Sheraton Hotel in Auckland. There were five award winners from different areas, including former New Zealand cricket captain Lee Germon, and each of us had to speak for seven minutes. My speech was similar to the one I do now, but looser as I didn't have any notes and was making it up as I went along. But as someone said later, it was from the heart. While the other speakers stood at lecterns and read notes, I was standing on my trestles and although it was gimmicky compared to the other speeches, everybody thought it was a good idea.

I thought of the scaffolding because climbing up it was something I did every day at work, and people would think, 'How does he do that?' Also, at the SMI awards night I needed a stage as the usual platforms are a foot off the ground and you stand behind a lectern. If I was on that platform no one would see me, so I thought, 'How could I do something to make people see me, and get a bit of attention?' Hence the trestles.

The reaction to my speech was tremendous — people stood up when I was finished and clapped. It was an awesome experience — people giving me a standing ovation. Me! Tony Christiansen, a signwriter from Tauranga. And hey, they didn't give Lee Germon, a former New Zealand cricket captain, a standing ovation. But Lee did win that night, and part of the prize was to go to America with SMI. Sure, I was disappointed that I didn't win — remember, I'm very competitive — and I felt that Lee's win was because everyone knew who he was and no one had heard of me.

After the speeches people came up and told me how good my speech was. Among them was Jim Hainey from Speakers New Zealand. As I was talking to Jim, well-known New Zealand comedian Mark Hadlow came up to me and said, 'Bloody brilliant, bloody brilliant, they picked the wrong winner.' That recognition gave me confidence. Jim gave me his card and said I now had an opportunity to become a speaker. I had never really thought about it before. I had heard speakers, of course, but didn't really know what they did. All I did was tell a story. I gave Jim a call because I thought I'd give it a go and I was never one to let an opportunity go by. Although Jim was enthusiastic about me, nothing happened as far as getting me some speaking work, which was disappointing, but I was glad I had tried.

New Zealand author and journalist Paul Smith contacted me and asked me if he could use my story as a chapter in his 1997 book, *Success in New Zealand Business II*, because of my signwriting business. Included in the book would be John Hart, then one of the most successful rugby coaches in New Zealand; media personality Paul Holmes, who not only hosted a national radio talkback show but a top-rating evening television current affairs show; young entrepreneur Stefan Lepionka, who started his own fresh orange juice business; computer business owner Sharon Hunter and internationally recognised playwright Roger Hall.

Then there was me — a signwriter from Tauranga. Of course I said yes.

Although Paul Smith focused on my business achievements, he also covered my sporting achievements, which were an important part of my life. I was invited to the book launch, presented by the publisher in association with the Auckland Chamber of Commerce, at the Aotea Centre. About four hundred people were there, and I was asked to speak for ten minutes about my life. Again, I used my trestles. And again I was given a standing ovation. I thought that was pretty cool. People thought enough of what I said to stand up and applaud — that was the most amazing thing for me.

Debbie Tawse from Celebrity Speakers New Zealand was at the book launch and no sooner had I got down from the trestles than she came up to me and said I'd be a good speaker for her and to give her a call.

So, of course, I did.

This time I hit success. Debbie told me she had a job for me in Rotorua if I was interested — at a Beaurepaires' sales and training conference. Naturally, I agreed. The conference was run by Robb Webb, who I went to school with, and he wanted me to speak for twenty minutes to the sales staff — two talks one day and one the next. I did a bit of a motivational speech to the staff and they loved it. Celebrity Speakers heard that I did okay. And the news reached further afield, because the next thing I had Jim Hainey ringing me to say he had some work for me.

From there my career as a speaker started. In 1998 I did fifty speaking jobs, in 1999 over eighty and it continues to grow. I am now getting frequent bookings in Australia, as well as speaking engagements in America. I am probably one of the most successful inspirational speakers in New Zealand today and I can't believe it. A lot of people can't believe it. It doesn't happen often, especially in New Zealand. But that goes to prove that if you set goals and try your hardest to succeed, then you will. It proved my point that you should take every opportunity that comes your way.

To some people, what I strived for was just a dream and hey, everyone's allowed to dream, they'd say, but really we should buckle down and get on with life — pay the mortgage, stay in a secure job, don't rock the boat. Count down to death. Well, I reckon that way of thinking is wrong. There is nothing wrong with dreaming, we all did it as kids, didn't we? When we grew up we wanted to be fire fighters or astronauts, princesses (well, not me) and pilots. Sure, those are dreams, but why shouldn't they come true? Because people dissuade us when we get older. 'Don't be silly, you can't be an astronaut, find yourself a sensible job.' People did that with me — 'You can't be a signwriter, you don't have any legs.'

We shouldn't destroy our kids' dreams. When you look at the world and all the amazing achievers — the Wright brothers, Albert Einstein — they were all dreamers once. And look what happened to their dreams. The same applies to adults. If one of your mates has got a dream, why should you impose your opinions on them — you never know, they could succeed. People said I couldn't fly or do Tae Kwon Do, but I did both.

I think that motivation of mine started when I was very young.

Ever since I could walk, I've always been on the go. I was a terror as a young child because I'd run away all the time. When I got older, I spent all my time hanging around with my friends so Mum never knew where I was. Even these days I have to be on the move, I really can't spend hours lying around doing nothing. I find it hard to stop — I'm always on the go. That's probably why I don't often read newspapers, because I'd have to stop and sit still for a while. Instead, I have to keep doing something, to keep moving.

I was once told at a self-improvement course that, with setting goals, once you have achieved what you set out to do and finished it, you've failed. That can be hard to get your head around at first, but it does make sense. I explain it this way — once you stop striving to do something, you've failed. Instead, you should always keep setting goals, achieving them and making sure you have another one after it, and another one after that. Keep on pushing yourself.

My brush with death when I was younger made me appreciate life so much more. I need my days to stand for something, everything has got to mean something, to be a step forward instead of wasting time on the mundane tasks in life. I believe procrastination is the killer of all people — if you're sitting around on your bum all day, what's that achieving? Nothing. (Although come to think of it, I'm sitting on my bum all the time — well, there goes that theory. Yikes!)

I was once told that if you stay in the same house for years, you're going backwards. If you've just moved home, you may disagree. My family and I have just had the drama of moving into our newly built house — we sold our old home and the new one wasn't ready on time so we had to bunk down at Elaine's dad's for a couple of months. Selling your house, buying a new one and then moving can be stressful, but it can be seen as being motivating — you're getting out there, pushing your boundaries, moving out of your comfort zones and the security of the house you have known for years. It's challenging because you're not stagnating in the same house year after year.

With that theory, maybe I should become a real estate agent.

But day-to-day I rush around. I always want to get out and do something with my day, I can't sit around at home and read a book. In the morning I can fly my plane, in the afternoon I can go jetskiing. I could be home by 3 p.m. watching television, and I'd be fidgeting around. So Elaine would kick me out of the house. 'Just go out and do something,' she'd say. It's like mowing the lawns at our place. I have a ride-on mower and I love cutting the lawns with it. I love getting out there and doing something, achieving something. We're going to have the shortest lawns in Tauranga.

My new career as an inspirational speaker makes the most of my need to keep moving. Recently I talked at a conference in Rotorua on a Friday morning, flew to Christchurch at midday, and caught a plane to Melbourne in the early afternoon. I spoke at Geelong, an hour south of Melbourne, that night, and then the next day headed back to Melbourne to fly to Sydney. I arrived there in the afternoon and on Saturday evening I set up my equipment. On Sunday I spoke at a conference. I flew back to Auckland on Monday, arrived late in the evening, and drove home to Tauranga. The next day, it was back to Auckland for another speech.

Phew! It was like, it's Sunday so this must be Sydney.

But I loved it, I really loved it. It kept me going, having to keep on my toes — so to speak — and push myself.

I always like to be as professional as I can. You want me in Melbourne on Friday? No problem. Instead of, 'Well, I'll be in Rotorua so I don't know if I can get a flight . . .' It doesn't matter, I'm motivated enough to agree to it, then find a flight to Melbourne. It's not such a big deal, there will always be a plane leaving for Australia somewhere in New Zealand. Besides, I certainly rake up the air points.

Elaine knows I'm good at public speaking and she's seen me at a couple of big seminars, but initially she was worried about whether I could support the family with my new career. In her eyes it was a big risk to sell the business and hope that I could make a career out of speaking. Luckily, she had faith in me and knew that I was determined enough to make it happen. She's known me long enough to realise that, once I set my mind to do something, I'll try my hardest to not only make it happen, but to do the very best I can. So though Elaine was petrified because I didn't have a regular income any more after selling Commercial Signs and quitting as an adviser, I was excited.

I felt my new career was only going to be as big as I made it. I looked at it like any business — if you didn't do your job you didn't get paid for it, and if you didn't produce what you said you would, you wouldn't get paid either. *I* am now the product. Whereas before I was selling signs, I am now selling Tony Christiansen. I have to make my product as professional as possible. I have created a website, www.tonytalks.com and it is an effective tool for reaching clients and letting people contact me. The website lists my achievements — after-dinner speaker; second-degree black belt; surf lifesaver; successful businessman; world class athlete; inspirational motivator; race car champion; qualified pilot; infotainer. I am proud of that résumé.

I've also included my favourite inspirational sayings on my website — like 'Positivity is its own motivation' and 'Your attitude dictates your attitude to life' — sayings that I hope will invigorate anyone who has seen me in action.

Letters from clients — both small groups and big corporations — are here, too. Those responses include: 'The feedback I received on your talk certainly reinforced my thoughts on the impact I hoped you would make. HUGE!' from Lion Breweries national sales training manager, Geoff Williamson.

'You just keep getting better and better! Not only do you have a real story to tell and the ability to tell it in a way that reaches everyone in the audience, but you also have the scores on the board to show it's how we respond to things that affect us that really matters,' from Dr Neil Flanagan, international best-selling author.

'Tony captured everyone's heart and passed on a very powerful message that totally embraced the essence of the whole conference which was, "seize the day",' from the Flight Centre's Auckland area manager, Michelle Sutton.

'Your session was undoubtedly the highlight of our two-day "Who Dares Wins" theme conference. The feedback and comments from our 60-plus attendees has been full of praise and positive comments for a great conference,' from Guardian Assurance's area manager, Pete J. Hobdell.

It makes me proud to read not only these letters but responses from ordinary people who have felt moved by what I have to say.

My full diary has reassured Elaine that I can make a go of my new career. I know that although my reputation as a top-class inspirational speaker is quickly building, that I must maintain that level and strive to be one of the best in the world.

And yes, I want to be wealthy, but not entirely for selfish reasons. I also want to make money to ensure that my family is provided for.

Sure, it may seem daunting at times — speaking at the SMI awards night, then the book launch, was a big step up for me from Rotary in Tauranga. But if I didn't give it a go then, I wouldn't be where I am today. And what was there for me to lose? Nothing. The biggest step was selling the business and having faith in myself, and from Elaine, that I could make speaking work my career.

I've never regretted selling Commercial Signs and becoming a speaker. Speaking is much less stressful than owning a business. A lot of people today tell you what you are doing wrong, but they don't tell you what you are doing right, and I found that in signwriting. The personal satisfaction had become less and less. My focus changed, I was working there at night doing my invoices and my staff were whingeing about wanting more money as they all thought I was making a million dollars. I didn't want that stress any more.

I decided at the start of my speaking career that I wanted to be a secret speaker — the audience wasn't to know that I was in a wheelchair. They might see the name Tony Christiansen and maybe the word 'pilot' but they shouldn't know about me not having any legs, and that works well because it creates that surprise element.

Okay, so I'm not cricket legend Richard Hadlee or someone that everyone knows. People have to come to one of my talks to hear what I've achieved and if you take away the fact that I don't have any legs they're still pretty good achievements and worth listening to. When you have the added challenge of being in a wheelchair then hopefully people are going to sit up and listen — and they do. I want to show that they aren't the only ones with challenges in their lives. I often outline the story of the accident, take them on an emotional roller coaster, and then leave them with a few thoughts.

When people read my résumé and see 'qualified pilot', 'black belt Tae Kwon Do' — they think I'm seven foot tall and bulletproof. Then I come out in a wheelchair, and people go, 'He can't be a pilot.' Then my credibility kicks in. How many speakers have you seen who stand behind the podium wearing a suit and tie and say, 'I'm successful, I'm a millionaire be- cause I've done this and this and this . . .'? I don't need to say that I don't have any legs and I can climb the ladder, because I go and do it.

People want to know my story — they want to know how I lost my legs. And that's the emotional roller coaster. I've had women crying in the front row because they're mothers. I've had men cry. When companies hire me they want to know my credibility, my success in business and what I'm going to talk about. When I speak, not only do I tell my story but I also try to tell the audience things they may not want to hear — things that make them question their life and achievements. But I'm not trying to motivate anyone. That word 'motivation' is a tough one. I don't like to think that I'm a motivational speaker; I'm an inspirational speaker. I'm really telling a story and hop- ing that listeners will be inspired enough by it to make a difference or make a change in their lives. Who knows the right way or the wrong way to live? I believe that our lives aren't scripted. I believe that we can do anything we want to. We just have to want to do it badly enough. We all have choices. We all have challenges in our lives — it's how we deal with them that matters. And I like to make challenges.

I also talk about adversity. They say that adversity makes you a better person, that a tragedy or a challenge in our life makes us dig down deep and brings out the best in us. So why are most of us sitting around waiting for something to happen before we go out and be the best we can be? There are people who have planned their lives so they've lessened the opportunity for adversity to hit; what they don't reckon on is that thing called fate. And when it does hit — inevitably — what are you going to do about it?

Why not just get out there and achieve?

I really believe that if you don't enjoy it, don't do it. I don't watch horror movies. I hate horror movies — I can't think of anything worse than having the heck scared out of me, so I don't watch them.

I suppose you can say that I've had a second chance. Instead of sitting around and dwelling on the things I'm never going to do, like being an All Black, I've gone out and done the things I can do. We all have choices, everyone has choices. Be they good or bad, it's what we make out of them. In my life, that attitude is what's taken me to where I am today — because I believe I can do it. If I had a dollar for every time I was told I couldn't do something in my life, I'd be a millionaire by now.

I've had people come up to me and say, 'Motivate me, I need motivation.' I can't motivate them. All I can do is inspire them to make a difference. You have a choice, just like I have. I have fewer choices than you have, but people think I have more. How do you work that one out?

I believe I have the potential to be one of the leading inspirational speakers in the world and I believe the only one who can make that happen is me. That is what I try to pass on during my speeches — no one else can make your goals happen, only you. And the reaction from people after my seminars differs. I've got lots of letters from people saying my speech changed their life. But they all get different messages. I spoke at a conference a while ago and a woman came up to me afterwards and said, 'I feel so inadequate, I may as well give up now.'

I was disappointed in myself, because I don't want to make anyone feel inadequate. I'm really trying to show them that with focus, with an attitude and a passion about the things you do, you can succeed. I kept thinking, 'What did I say in my presentation to make her think that?' So I asked her why she felt inadequate.

She said, 'I'm thirty-eight years old and I haven't achieved anything.'

'You're maybe not going to achieve these things. The reason I've achieved these things is because I want to. It's as simple as that,' I said to her.

The woman said, 'I want to do some things.'

'Do you believe you can do them?' I asked.

'I've never really thought about it that much,' was her reply.

I told her, 'Never feel inadequate because of anything I've said. You should really look to what you believe, because it's not about me, it's about you. All I'm trying to do is inspire you by showing you that even with the physical challenge in my life I'm able to achieve the things I do. But I do it because I want to do it. What are the things you want to do?'

She couldn't answer me.

It's all about perception. It's about perception of ourselves and it's about the perception other people have of us. So I said to her, 'Until you can find a way, don't feel inadequate, because that's your mental perception of you. You're the only one who can make a difference. I can only enthuse you or inspire you to make a difference. Whether you do or not is completely up to you. So never feel inadequate.'

I then asked her if she was happy.

She replied, 'Yeah, most of the time.'

I said, 'Then why do you feel inadequate?'

'Because I haven't achieved as much as you.'

I said, 'Hello! Haven't you been listening? It's about choice. Where in the script does it say you have to be as good as Tony Christiansen? That you have to do the same things he's done?'

She said, 'It doesn't.'

So she answered her own question.

But I've also had some memorable positive feedback. A woman rang me and said she had struggled to find me but she had to track me down as her son had been at one of my conferences. He was 17 years old and up until that time he had no direction in his life. In the two weeks since my speech he'd made a total turnaround. He kept talking about 'Tony this' and 'Tony that'. He was so inspired but he didn't know where he could find a small book written for children that I sold at my seminars. So she went around town looking for the book, but she couldn't find it anywhere. She asked me if I would give her a book and sign it, because I had inspired her son so much. I suggested that her son and I get together some time so we could talk some more, and I sent him the book with the inscription: 'Life will only give you want you ask for, nothing more, nothing less. Ask wisely.'

I think the major challenge facing some young people is that they don't know what they want or what they would like to do. Sometimes it's best not to give them the answers — that's the easy way out — but rather to show them the choices they have. Ask questions and get them to think and so discover the answers for themselves. It's too easy to tell people what they should or shouldn't do; and what would they learn, anyway? That's why I love talking to schools — to try to inspire kids who are at such an important stage of their lives.

I talked at a luncheon meeting a while ago and a woman from Rotorua, Deborah Bell, thought my presentation would be ideal for high school kids. I spoke to the six high schools in Rotorua and I aimed to give a low-key speech; I tried to talk to them rather than lecture them. The response was great. I got heaps of letters from the classes and it was fantastic to receive feedback, especially from the 13–14 year old girls, because I think they are going to have the hardest time in their life. A lot of them believe they don't have many options, so I tried to show them that they did.

Other speeches I have given are memorable for their location or the size of the audience. A chain of video stores, Video Ezy, held a seminar in Fiji for its New Zealand and Australian franchise owners and I spoke there. It was fantastic, although it was hard to concentrate in such a beautiful location.

But my largest, most phenomenal seminar to date, was the conference for the Interactive Distribution Association, a part of Amway, at the Mystery Creek centre near Hamilton. I spoke to 4500 people — my largest audience — and I received a standing ovation. Image that — 4500 people standing up and applauding me. It was pretty daunting when I first went on stage as I had a spotlight on me and could only see a few rows of people in the front. Although it is usually hard to interact with a large group, the Amway crowd was pretty enthusiastic to start with.

Elaine had decided she wanted to watch me speak at IDA. She had planned to come to my speech, but all the accommodation in Hamilton was booked out and I had to bunk in with one of the organisers. Of course I was disappointed, as this was going to be my biggest audience yet, but I left Tauranga for Hamilton thinking Elaine wouldn't be there. Half an hour later Elaine got in her car and followed me, but her plan to surprise me nearly came unstuck. She'd just got out of her car at the car park at the convention centre and could hear the crowd inside clapping and yelling at another speaker, when I rang her on her cell phone.

I said, 'Can you hear this lot?'

Elaine was thinking to herself, 'Yeah, I can hear it in stereo' but instead she said to me, 'It sounds like a really enthusiastic crowd.' She then wished me well and told me I'd do a good job.

As I went on stage Elaine went to the back door, and was let backstage when she said she was my wife. She was very impressed with my speech but was slightly annoyed when I said I had been married for over twenty years and was applauded. She felt she deserved the applause, not me!

After the high of speaking in front of 4500 people, the next day I went to the opposite extreme, talking to just 24 people at a meeting for a group of insurance people. So I had to change my tack and try to interact with them more.

To end my speeches I usually smash three wooden boards set up on metal stands. It's an impressive conclusion, the bang of the wood breaking. I do it to make an impact, a statement about obstacles and breaking through mental barriers. When I do smaller seminars I get other people to smash the boards, because most of the time people think it's impossible. When I pick women to break the boards, they usually say they can't do it. But I tell them, 'Come on, this is for you, this is your chance, your time now.' I talk about it with them, make them touch the board, focus on the board. All the time I'm holding the board and bending and twisting it to show them this solid object. I make them concentrate and then get them to hit the board. They think they are going to break their knuckles. But you build these people up and then BANG, when they hit it, the board smashes in the middle. Of course, what they don't realise is that when I'm bending the board I'm making it weak in the middle. That doesn't matter, the fact, is they did it.

I like to make a big impact with my speech, and a positive side of being up on stage is being able to give something back. I've had a lot of great opportunities and some fantastic people have helped me, so I want to help people too. When my time comes I want my life to stand for something. It doesn't matter if someone has changed their life because of something I've spoken about or because they've read this book, I'm just glad they decided to do something about their life. What I love to hear after my speeches is that people are looking at themselves and their life in a different way. That things aren't as bad as they think, that they've had some adversity in their life and I've helped them change the way they see either themself or those around them. I've talked to thousands of people through my speaking and had some great feedback. Some people leave my seminar not thinking much about it, but that's okay, because everyone is going to see what I do differently. It's great to have the opportunity to make a difference to people's lives. I'm the type of person who likes to touch, likes to feel his work. I used to be very proud of what Commercial Signs did. There was always that sense of achievement in seeing your work out there, and that's what I look for — that feedback. It makes me feel really good and it's an important part of my work.

A big part of my work is the preparation for an event. When I get to a venue I talk to the venue management about my set-up and usually the local Projex Hire Company has delivered my scaffolding. The trestle is set up and if I've driven to the venue then I change in the back of my Ford van. Sometimes I have to fly in for a conference and stay in a hotel, and that can be boring for a 'hyperactive' person like me. But I am being paid to be a professional so I make sure that I am well prepared for each speaking engagement.

As I have a concept and story the way I tell it may be different every time. The contents are the same, it's just how I feel at the time and how I feel the audience is going to respond on the night. I don't tell jokes, I tell stories. The stories are humorous and they convey my message but they also say, 'Hey, Tony is real as well — he laughs.' I'm not trying to be a comedian, I'm just using humour to emphasise my point.

I have to be a performer, an entertainer, because it is difficult to keep people's attention for an hour if they're not being entertained. You have to try to gain their respect and I usually do that with interaction. You can't interact with 4500 people, but interacting with a small group is easily done just by asking questions: 'Come on, how many of you are goal setters?'

A spin-off from my speaking was a children's literacy book about me written by Angie Belcher. Her husband was a signwriter in Tauranga and out of the blue Angie rang me. She wrote for Learning Media children's books and she thought I'd be a great subject and wanted to know if I'd be interested. She said it wouldn't be profitable for me but it would be a great opportunity. I agreed, and Learning Media subsequently published *The Sky's The Limit*. It became one of Learning Media's best sellers. I attended the book launch in Auckland and there I met Anna Kenna, a reporter with TV3's '20/20' television programme, who also wrote children's books. She was keen to do a story on me. When she showed my book to her producer he said, 'Go for it.' So Anna and the '20/20' crew came to Tauranga for three days to film my family and me. It was pretty intensive — shooting me in the swimming pool and in my plane — but it was very interesting to see how such programmes worked.

The media has taken an interest in me since the first days of my accident. When I was involved in motor sports I was often interviewed because I was a novelty. I have been on

'Deaker Profiles', Sky television's half-hour sports interview show with Murray Deaker, plus I've had a guest spot on Mary Lambie's 'Good Morning' on TV One, as well as a couple of appearances on the Holmes show. I've also had numerous radio interviews and recently had my first go at talkback. I was being interviewed — for what I thought would be fifteen minutes — and it turned into nearly an hour with listeners phoning in and asking me questions. I was quite nervous at first and found it hard to have a conversation with a microphone, but then I began to enjoy it and loved chatting to the listeners.

The media attention is good as it enables people to learn about me and it gives me confidence to aim towards my next goal — being one of the best speakers in the world. I know that I can do it. I am over the stage shock, it doesn't daunt me any more, and I could easily speak to 10,000 or even 50,000 people if I had to. It would be pretty cool. I suppose it's the showman in me coming out. I want to be an entertainer and that's why I'm busy now. The opportunities are there for me at present, from speaking at business conferences and seminars to overseas work. But while there are quite a few speakers on the circuit, I don't think there is a lot of work for all of them. The big names — like cricket legends Sir Richard Hadlee and Jeremy Coney — get the work because of their fame in their sport. I'm an unknown, however, so I'm proud and pleased to be so busy.

> *Jim Hainey, owner of Speakers New Zealand, has been a speaker both in New Zealand and Australia and has owned the company since 1994. The company was established in 1984.*

When I saw Tony speak at the SMI awards night his presentation was pretty raw, but he had the makings of a sincere person

— someone who genuinely believed in themselves. What I liked about Tony was that he was a real down-to-earth Kiwi. I thought people could relate to him.

Tony has a very likeable manner and a good sense of humour. There was a lot of humour in his presentation — much of it was accidental and spontaneous.

At the end of his speech, he said he had a dream to become an inspirational speaker and I'm a big fan of people having dreams. I gave him my card and said that he should give me a call if he wanted to pursue speaking. I eventually went to see him in Tauranga and from there we developed a more polished presentation and smoothed the edges out a little bit. He presented his story in a very positive way.

It takes many different qualities to become a good speaker. You have to be genuine, and have commitment to the story. You need to have something that will change people's lives. You need to have a certain character, a certain integrity. You need to be adding, not subtracting from the audience. And you need to be doing it for the message rather than for the money. People with a story don't have to be great speakers, they just need to have a story and tell it with passion.

Tony is a storyteller in the best possible way — he tells his story, about his obvious so-called disability, and he tells people how he overcame it. He's very inspiring.

Tony would be one of the top three speakers in New Zealand and maybe in the top five or six in Australia. Internationally, he's probably in the top ten or fifteen.

A lot of speaking has to do with marketing. If Tony had an unlimited audience flow, people could well consider him one of the best speakers in the world. But you need to get the audiences in front of you and New Zealand is not necessarily the best place to get a hundred and fifty presentations a year.

There are some fine speakers in the world. The best of

them take you on a journey, and by the end of their talk your life has changed forever. That is what Tony does.

There's a certain attitude in Australia and New Zealand — the just-get-on-and-do-it approach — that I think contributes to the type of people we are. The Americans, and the English to a lesser extent, think it's quite remarkable that someone in Tony's position just gets on with it and doesn't sit in the background. Tony has a boyishness about him and people like the fact that he's one of the boys. People can relate to him; they think, 'Wow, he's just like me except I've got legs and he hasn't.' He's quite infectious and as long as he doesn't lose that then I think the Americans will love him.

> *Debbie Tawse* is the owner of Celebrity Speakers (NZ). She has thirteen years experience in the industry, over ten years in her own business.

I was very impressed with Tony when I heard him speak at the *Success in New Zealand Business II* book launch. I really thought he was great, I knew that he had it. I couldn't stop at the launch to talk to him so I gave him my card, got his number and I phoned him immediately. I was prepared to drive to Tauranga to see Tony as I was so impressed with him; it's not very often that I'd phone someone up and say I'll drive to see you. I just don't do that with speakers.

He made an impact on me because here was a guy who got on with life, was prepared to talk about his experiences and could laugh at himself. At the time, because he was green and inexperienced, he was very, very natural.

One of the challenges for us is that people are always looking for a new speaker. So when we have a good speaker who is new, that's who the clients want and that's been the case with Tony.

The thing that makes a good speaker is how much they can change their story, how many different speeches they can do. The way to have an extended 'shelf life' is to be able to come up with new things, to be able to change so it's not the same story that people hear all the time. Tony is determined to work at this, and I think that if people are prepared to develop and take advice then they can be successful. In his specific field, Tony is certainly one of the leading speakers in Australasia. He is out there doing a good job and getting a good number of bookings. He's sought after and he delivers.

I think it takes one of two things to become a successful speaker overseas. Profile really counts, international profile of the kind that Sir Edmund Hillary has. Jonah Lomu is huge in the UK but not so big in the States, because the USA is not traditionally a rugby nation. I'm talking huge, huge profile on top of being a good, articulate speaker. Otherwise, it takes someone who is a really good speaker, and who is prepared to work at his or her craft, to be in it for the long haul. They must know that nothing happens overnight, that moving into the US market is not a matter of a one-month or two-month job. It takes years to build into that world-class, huge market.

The sheer volume over there is different. You have to have instantaneous things — your own videos, your own website updated daily — and all of these things cost money. Because of the scale of fees in New Zealand, many of our speakers wouldn't have the budget to do the marketing that they need in the States. That's even the situation for a company like mine, and I am running one of the larger speaking bureaus. We're chipping away at it, but for a speaker to do it on their own, it takes a lot of work, a lot of money and a lot of time. You have to be very determined and you have to be very patient. Not everyone has that tenacity. But I think Tony is capable of being a world-class motivational speaker.

CHAPTER NINE
THE GOAL OF
GOALSETTING

*'Life is like driving a car, if you don't steer it you end
up going somewhere you don't want to be.'*

ALTHOUGH I've achieved many things in my life I never stop
setting goals. They may be big goals compared to some people's but I'm determined to make the most out of life. One of
the things I have in mind for the next few years is to circum-
navigate New Zealand solo in an aeroplane; that would make
New Zealand history as I'd be the first disabled pilot to do so.
I may also give flying trans-Tasman solo a try — that's his-
tory-making too. I'd love to snow ski and try the luge. I heard
there is a place in Europe that holds luge courses for the disabled, so I'm keen to pursue that.

It's simple enough to think of these goals — or dreams —
but it may seem daunting to achieve them. One of the major
parts of goal setting is having the dream or vision in the first
place, and then working out the steps to realise that goal.

And for me, my goals come from the dreams I have — the
things that excite me, the things that are important in my life.

First, I sit down with a piece of paper and write what my
dream is; that is an important step. By committing your goal
to paper you make it real — you're no longer thinking, 'What

if?' instead you have something to work towards. Then, on the paper, I plan how I'm going to achieve that goal.

An important part of that is I look at life as a balance sheet: we all have assets and liabilities, that is, strengths and weaknesses. My assets are I'm a very enthusiastic person; I'm a good communicator; I have ways of creating money if I need it for my goal. For example, if the particular goal has some financial costs then I could look at my speaking to finance it, or I could do some signwriting after hours to earn some extra money, or I could sell something that I no longer need. Those are three simple ways I could go about financing my goal. Another asset is my 'never give up' attitude — I will do whatever it takes to make that goal come true.

On the other side are my liabilities — and we should think of the liabilities that we can control. For example, one liability could be the cost of my goal. I find out the cost at the start so I know if the goal is realistic. One of my liabilities could be my stubbornness. I try to fast-track some of the things that I need to do, rather than go step by step. By recognising that as a liability I can try to do something about it.

Once I have assessed my assets and liabilities I can formulate a plan that will allow me to work through and achieve my goal. For example, one of the goals I'm working on currently is learning how to snow ski and it's something that is very real — I can see it happening, I've got a vision and I know what I want to achieve. I decided I wanted to learn how to snow ski because it has always excited me. I've seen other people with physical disabilities doing it and because of things that I have done before, like water skiing, it's something I want to master. I'm not saying that I want to be the best in the world, but I want to master the art of snow skiing, to be self-sufficient at it.

Step one is to set the goal, step two is to work out your

assets and liabilities and the third step — and another important one — is to tell people your goal. By talking about your goal other people can share in it and give you feedback, enthusiasm and knowledge. It's a 'who you know' world. Through telling people my skiing goal I've found out that two friends involved in disabled sports also ski.

The next step is working out what I have to do to achieve it — and that includes making calls. I've found out there's a special ski that I can use. It costs about $800 and is made by an American company called Shadow. The ski is a lightweight steel frame with a seat on it that you strap around yourself and clip onto the ski. It has a shock-absorber in the cantilevered arm that acts like a knee-joint by coming forward and then back. An able-bodied skier keeps their knees bent and they act as suspension when you ski; the cantilevered arm does the same thing.

I also have to find a place to ski. Although I live in the North Island and there are ski fields nearby, we haven't had good snow seasons recently. And as most of the disabled skiing is done in the South Island I would probably have to travel to the southern ski resorts. This means it's not a cheap sport — I have to finance the ski, travel to Mt Hutt or Cardrona ski fields, pay for accommodation and ski passes, and then ski lessons. When I look at the cost involved I have to think if I can afford it. If I can't afford to do the whole thing, what parts can I afford to do this year?

So every day it's thinking about it, it's doing something like making a phone call, working out how much something costs. I believe we need to do something constructive every day of our lives — take those steps to become successful. Then we are doing three, four or five things a day simultaneously, but we don't recognise it sometimes. I believe everything has a flow-on effect. You do one thing, something else follows. But if you don't do anything, nothing else will follow. It's like the saying — life is like driving a car, if you don't steer it you end up going somewhere you don't want to be.

With my skiing goal, I have the following assets: my determination; I can generate the income to afford to do it; I know people who can teach me; and I have the opportunity to buy a ski through a friend. My liabilities are working it into my tight schedule as speaking is my priority; making sure my fitness is up to standard; finding snow; and that my timing fits in with the people who are going to teach me.

Disabled skiing is taught by a couple of able-bodied people who coach the New Zealand disabled skiing team. While my initial goal is to learn how to ski — and I've had a couple of goes at it before but never really knuckled down to it — I can also think ahead to representing New Zealand in the winter Paralympics.

It is a realistic goal but I think, with my speaking being the main thing in my life and my major goal of being a world-class speaker, that many of my other goals will have to take second place. And I've still got more mundane goals — like mowing the lawns.

Another one of my 'secondary' goals is circumnavigating New Zealand solo, so I apply the same principles to that. My assets include the fact that I'm a pilot; I can do cross-country flying; I could find people who would sponsor me financially; I know lots of people in the aviation area who are enthusiastic about helping me to achieve that goal. On the liabilities side there are the logistics of the whole thing; dealing with civil aviation's paperwork to get permission to do this; fitness; the weather; and fitting it in with my schedule.

Yet another goal of mine is to race a sprint car in Australia, and I've been speaking to people about this. My assets are that I have the experience to be able to race a sprint car; I know people involved in the sport; I can find the financial backing to do it. The liabilities are getting a car, either finding one in Australia or shipping one over from New Zealand; then if I do ship one over I must get the car from the wharf to the track; and there are many logistical problems.

In every one of my goals my biggest asset is my attitude and my willingness to work through the step-by-step planning stages.

Those are just three of my goals. I'm 41 years old and if I'm realistic about my sporting life, I've got only ten or fifteen years left in which I'm going to be physically able to do these things because I rely on my arms so much. So I have to make these things happen while I can.

If you are still unsure about the benefits of goal setting then look around you. There are many successful people in business, sports and entertainment and many of them have common qualities — they are goal setters, they are planners, dreamers and believers.

The recipe for success is simple. The hard part is taking the first step, the rest of it is easy.

Successful people are always busy. People may look at an achiever like Microsoft boss Bill Gates and think, 'He's got all those billions of dollars, he doesn't need to work.' But it's in the achievers' nature to work as they enjoy it so much and they are passionate about it. They will never settle for second best and they will never stop. That's what makes them successful. They want to keep achieving their goals, they want to keep doing things with their life.

Start thinking about your life and what you want out of it. Are you happy? Are you fulfilled? Are you passionate about something? Don't let barriers get in the way, like thinking, 'I can't do that because I have a family, or a mortgage.' We often put barriers in our way — and we have to look through them.

Never stop dreaming. Never let anyone take your dreams away. There are so many people out there who are willing to drag you down to their level instead of aspiring to yours.

We are in a world of endless possibilities, of endless opportunities.

When I think back to the Wright brothers achieving their dream of flight, when I think back to Thomas Edison and his dream of light, I realise that every great idea in this world has come from somebody's dream. You just have to believe in yourself. Believe in achieving your goals.

People say, 'Tony, how do you become so motivated? Where do you get this attitude? You can't go down the road and buy it.'

Motivation comes from the heart. I tell people, they took away my legs, but they didn't take my heart, they didn't take my passions, and they didn't take my desires. We live in a world where we are told that if you're not a winner, you're a loser. If you're not a success, you're a failure. We're given examples of this every day of our lives. We see it on the television, read it in the newspapers.

I don't believe that at all, it's not about winning or losing in this life, it's about how you play the game. It's about being the best you can be. Each one of us has the potential in our life to achieve greatness. We just have to believe in ourself. Believe who we are, believe what we stand for in our life. And this belief comes from having an attitude.

The world will only give you what you ask for, nothing more, nothing less. Be very sure about what you ask.